"Few events create fear in our beings like a diagnosis of brain disease. Ann's book reaches across that fear with warmth, knowledge, and practical wisdom. The strange world of medical mystery now has a guide from someone who has been there. Whether it is planning for your first MRI or hearing a gloomy prognosis, the book is a wise friend. It is the missing piece in patient care."

—Priscilla Ingebrigtsen, LCSW

"Ann's personal story reflects not only a living caregiver's perspective, but it also offers insights from her husband George about issues that only fellow brain tumor survivors can truly appreciate. This book is a heartfelt expression of the hope, faith, and love Ann and George have shared with each other throughout their brain tumor journey."

—Nancy Conn-Levin, M.A., Health Educator and Brain Tumor Survivor

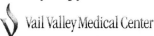

A Caregiver's Story

A Caregiver's Story

Coping with A Loved One's Life-Threatening Illness

Ann Brandt

iUniverse, Inc.
New York Lincoln Shanghai

A Caregiver's Story
Coping with A Loved One's Life-Threatening Illness

iUniverse books may be ordered through booksellers or by contacting:

iUniverse
2021 Pine Lake Road, Suite 100
Lincoln, NE 68512
www.iuniverse.com
1-800-Authors (1-800-288-4677)

Because of the dynamic nature of the Internet, any Web addresses or links contained in this book may have changed since publication and may no longer be valid.

The views expressed in this work are solely those of the author and do not necessarily reflect the views of the publisher, and the publisher hereby disclaims any responsibility for them.

ISBN: 978-0-595-44883-8 (pbk)
ISBN: 978-0-595-69539-3 (cloth)
ISBN: 978-0-595-89208-2 (ebk)

Printed in the United States of America

Weeping may tarry for the night,
but joy comes in the morning.

—Psalm 30:5

Contents

Introduction

In 1998, my husband, George, was diagnosed with primary CNS non-Hodgkin's lymphoma, a rare type of brain tumor. Doctors expected him to die within weeks. Instead, with the help of God and the medical community, he survived. I had just recovered from another little-known illness—Guillain Barre. As George had been my caregiver the previous year, I would become his caregiver in our battle against brain cancer.

In writing this book, I visualized the faces of men and women of all ages who come to our brain tumor support group for the first time. Most of them are in shock, just as I was when my husband was diagnosed with brain cancer. All of them want to see others who have been diagnosed with brain cancer; they need to listen and, later, to talk. I watch their expressions when the word *survivor* comes up. It is like throwing a life vest to a drowning person. They are hungry for hope. That's what I wish to offer here.

To battle cancer is to walk a long and difficult path, and coping with the effects of brain cancer adds an extra challenge. In this book, you will learn how my husband and I struggled to accept the changes that brain cancer forces on the lives of the person diagnosed as well as on friends and family. Brain cancer is unique from other types of cancer, because it affects the mind and emotions far more deeply. The tumors that invade the space that makes us who we are, our emotions and our intellect, steal from us in one degree or another. Moreover, as with any serious and life changing disease, we grieve for what is lost and we struggle to adapt.

A vital factor in survival is hope. Early in our cancer journey, my husband and I were given the gift of hope. The dictionary defines hope as desire accompanied by expectation, but hope is much more than that. Hope is the essential ingredient that holds the soul together. God embedded hope in us before we were born. Suffering, sharing, and surviving boils down to a quest for hope, the element with which humanity obtains its existence. When times get tough—illness, loss, end-of-life issues for us and for our loved ones—suffering people come together and share hope as one would share food or water with the hungry or thirsty. Hope sometimes strengthens courage to face the fact that the will of God prevails over our desire for control. Hope gives us the faith to know that whatever trials we endure, God is there with us during the black times.

The term "walking through the fire" best describes a cancer journey. I have seen people endure pain and suffering beyond imagining, emerging stronger in spirit. The time of my husband's illness was such an experience, one that brought out strengths I did not know I possessed.

I knew without question that it would be my turn to care for him as he had cared for me, and that I would dedicate myself to his wellbeing as fully as he had mine. The enormity of our situation and the reality of our mortality ran over me like a tank. I was plunging into the biggest task of my life, without tools or instructions. However, I remembered how my husband had taken care of me, lovingly and completely, and I vowed to let that experience be my blueprint for caregiving.

This book is intended to share the things I learned during my husband's battle to survive. You will hear my voice, my point of view, expressing and explaining as I share with you the things I learned during that summer of what we now call "the cancer." Caring for a person with brain tumors carries demands not present in taking care of people with other types of cancer. Surviving brain cancer requires special coping techniques. You will read a first-person account of how my husband came back from what he calls his "dark place" of confusion and helplessness.

The body and the mind are both affected by brain tumors. I have seen brain tumor patients whose emotions are fragile, vacillating from sad to happy and back again in the space of a few minutes. Loved ones need to know how to deal with emotional storms. Brain tumors are another form of brain injury, so recovery involves rebuilding mind as well as body. Everyone's cancer journey is unique, and there are many ways to cope with the changes in mind and body during treatment and afterward.

Some brain tumors are non-malignant (or benign). They are no less destructive to brain tissue and surrounding areas, and they carry the possibility of becoming malignant. In our brain tumor support group we have seen patients with benign brain tumors endure everything that cancer patients suffer: uncertainty, pain, cognitive issues, and physical changes.

The brain cancer experience of my husband and me included prayer, angels, spiritual healing, and medical expertise. We consider each ingredient vitally important. Immediately after he was diagnosed, my husband asked everyone he knew to pray for him, that his life would be prolonged so that he and I might enjoy just a little more time together. I prayed to eliminate the feeling of isolation as I saw my companion of many years lose his personality in a confusion of garbled speech and disorientation.

George was quite deteriorated mentally and physically by the time he entered cancer treatment. Through a series of errors and misjudgments, a correct diagnosis was delayed until he was unable to speak, understand, or even move without harming himself. Later, however, we learned that the delay saved his life, as you will read here.

At one point during the intense chemotherapy treatments, side effects attacked with such pain that George asked the Lord to take him then. That didn't happen. Instead, there appeared one more of a succession of what we now call angels on Earth to advise, encourage, pray, and offer hope. I offer this book as an angel on Earth for you and for your loved ones.

Chapter 1
The Journey Begins

The words that change a life more than any other are, "You have brain cancer." For years, cancer and death have linked to create a terror that defies description. I had always associated brain cancer with dying. My only knowledge of brain cancer had included images of hollow-eyed people with hideous scars on hairless heads. These imaginations were obviously fed by fear. Brain cancer, I always told myself, was something that happened to other people. It would never happen to me or to anyone I loved. But it did. I'll never forget the day I looked at an image that even to my unpracticed eye announced that something was wrong with my husband's brain.

After the shock came fear. For a few awful moments, I felt my husband drifting away into a world that I could not enter. Feelings of fear and hopelessness can be as harmful and hard to overcome as the actual cancer. The shock and panic brought by a diagnosis of cancer is usually the first obstacle to overcome. The person with the tumor will be the central figure in this cancer journey, but others will play important parts as well.

After our session with the oncologist, we walked across the parking lot, unmindful of the warm spring breeze, in stunned silence. We sat in the car, speechless for what seemed like hours. I thought of our four children; adults with families of their own, they all lived in various parts of the country. Imagining their shock upon hearing about their father's cancer, I shrank from the idea of calling them.

My husband was unable to help because of his condition, and I was almost as helpless because of my shock. Then, as my husband and I had always done in crisis, we began forming a battle plan. Neither one of us had ever lapsed into inaction in the face of adversity. George had always been the one to focus on the specific problem and research a solution, but this time problem solving would be up to me. A cold, empty feeling washed over me as I realized the responsibility being thrust on me. For the first time in our married lives, I was the strong one, the person responsible for making decisions and initiating actions. I felt very lonely.

The oncologist had suggested that we find a "good neurosurgeon." Where does one find such a person? I wondered. Where would we start? We would need to call on others for help and advice for this first step. At this point, the tumors had not been officially identified. We knew only that four large "masses" dominated the space in the middle of George's brain. Only later, far into the cancer journey, did I learn about the various types of brain tumors and survival statistics on each type.

The most common primary brain tumor type is meningioma, a benign tumor that has all the risks of malignant tumors. Glioblastoma multiforme, a malignant tumor, is the second most common type. In our support group, many of the patients have been diagnosed with GBMs. It is believed that there are two types of GBMs. One type starts as a low-or intermediate-grade astrocytoma and progresses to grade IV, thus becoming a glioblastoma multiforme. Dr. Vinay Puduvalli, assistant professor and director of the fellowship program of neuro-oncology at M. D. Anderson in Houston, Texas, says, "The other type, known as a denovo form, seems to start out as a glioblastoma. This division seems to be due to differences in the genetic changes that trigger the growth of these tumors." In other words, the tumor was a GBM to start with. In the late 1990s, many of the treatments used today had not been FDA approved. Some medications, such as Temador, were just coming into clinical trials. Research on identifying tumor subtypes and on creating and customizing new treatment plans and medicines continues as the survival rate on all brain tumors rises steadily.

George's tumor type was considered rare in 1998 and remains in the minority of brain tumor occurrences. The Central Brain Tumor Registry of the United States (CBTRUS) states that lymphomas of the brain account for only 3 percent of all primary brain tumors as of 2004. Primary central nervous system non-Hodgkin's lymphoma is a long title that defines lymphoma in the brain. Researching this tumor put me on two paths—reading material describing lymphoma and studying the more general subject of brain cancer. This form of cancer occurs when cells from a body's immune system grow out of control. For that reason, George had to undergo a spinal tap and bone marrow test in addition to blood tests to determine absence of AIDS before doctors would begin crafting a treatment plan.

The attending physician was a hematologist/oncologist—a physician specializing in diseases of the blood as well as cancer—and the doctor working with her under the hospital fellowship program was outstanding in his compassionate manner. Dr. Schultz explained our options for treatment, once he saw the biopsy results. We could opt for radiation, he explained, or George could undergo strong chemotherapy. The effects of radiation, however, would result in severe deficits—physical and cognitive. How long, we wanted to know, could George live. Dr. Schultz drew a deep breath, observing our expectant expressions. "With immediate treatment, people live a couple of years, at best. Twelve weeks most probable, if he survives the treatment."

Since that day, I have often thought of how hard it must be for a doctor to give such news to patients and their families, who present themselves in front of a trained specialist, hoping against all odds that this professional, with all of his or her knowledge and training, can make everything all right. Sometimes, I wonder if that's why we see so many physicians who appear cold and uncaring—perhaps they are in fact protecting themselves from emotional overspending that will sap their energies.

Dr. Schultz, however, managed to combine compassion with skill. He promised to bring me some written material on the subject of radiation and survival rates. He opened the door to leave, then turned around and said softly, "I'll pray for you." We clung to those words and will never forget them or him.

When I read the statistics in the material Dr. Schultz brought later that day, panic enveloped me once again. According to the literature, many people diagnosed with CNS lymphoma also have AIDS. With treatment and without the presence of AIDS, a person could live 18.9 months. I realize now that those figures were published from data compiled five years previously and that survival rates were then, as now, constantly increasing. It does not help patients or their caregivers to obsess on survival rates shown on a chart compiled from data gathered five years earlier. What matters is *your* survival. I decided that for my own mental health, I would not dwell on survival rates displayed in charts. I advise you to avoid thinking about charts showing survival rates.

I learned by talking to several medical personnel and by researching on the Internet that CNS lymphoma tumors are slow growing, responsive to treatment, and often present with multiple tumors. George had four well-defined masses on his MRI. In 1998, many new drugs and methods were still in clinical trials, so we were told that CNS lymphomas invariably return soon after remission, and with great ferocity. For the first year after being pronounced cancer free, we lived under a cloud of uncertainty. Doctors told George to "get his affairs in order," a phrase that was repugnant to me. However, instead of waiting for the other shoe to drop, as the expression goes, my husband and I now live each day as if it is the last one we have together. At the same time, we freely make long-term plans and look forward to the future, however long it may be. Since our battle with brain cancer in 1998, the drug Rituxan has been approved and is now used both as a front-line medication for CNS lymphoma and as part of treatment for recurrent tumors. I look upon the drug as a kind of safety net.

In the first months after George's diagnosis, and especially during that crucial first year of recovery when everything seemed so uncertain, I read much of the material from the three national brain tumor groups: American Brain Tumor Association, the Brain Tumor Society, and the National Brain Tumor Foundation. Each one offers information and support to patients, families, and medical professionals

The American Brain Tumor Association publishes a comprehensive booklet that describes each of the many types of brain tumors—malignant and benign—including tumors occurring in children. The booklet also explains in general terms the various types of treatments. You can obtain a copy of *A Primer of Brain Tumors* from the address listed in the appendix.

While the rate of primary malignant brain tumors of all kinds is increasing—forty thousand in 2004—survival rates are also on the rise. New treatments are constantly being developed, as well as advanced diagnostic methods. New methods to reduce the side effects of treatment also allow patients to endure a full course of treatment with fewer brutal side effects, whereas, years ago, many people undergoing cancer medication would opt out of treatment, essentially giving up the will to live. In today's society, we are turning away from the long-held notion that a cancer diagnosis is a death sentence.

The First Signs of a Brain Tumor

When you look back on the days preceding your diagnosis, it's natural to think about symptoms that fit into a pattern, like pieces of a puzzle—jumbled until you arrange them into a recognizable picture. Part of the diagnostic process involves sorting out and categorizing your symptoms, often using a process of elimination. You and your physician are partners in this stage, and you will remain in close communication throughout your cancer journey. Doctors need all the information they can garner. This is where your caregiver and loved ones can be a big help. They have observed you and perhaps noted any changes, however gradual, that have occurred over the past weeks or months. Sometimes it is easier for others to notice changes in our physical abilities, because it is natural for most people to adjust unconsciously to physical limitations as they develop.

If you and your loved ones can sort through symptoms and put a timeline on them, you will be able to give your physician valuable information. Physicians must be detectives, problem solvers, and scientists all at once in this most important stage—the diagnosis. Taken separately, no unusual occurrence may signal that something is wrong. Yet several of these symptoms should mean a call for help.

Maybe there was a persistent headache that started every morning but seemed to go away as the day went on. Nausea and vomiting can sometimes signal the presence of a brain tumor, but queasiness will also occur with stomach upset or gastrointestinal infection. Dizziness and loss of balance can be symptoms of inner ear infection, anemia, or hypoglycemia, or half a dozen other maladies. Memory loss and inability to think quickly or clearly can manifest so gradually that a person doesn't notice or learn to compensate. Those symptoms can also be attributed to many conditions, such as menopause, hypothyroid, fatigue, or stress.

A word about stress: don't let your physician throw out a general blanket of stress as a diagnosis. There are two disadvantages to accepting a diagnosis of stress. First, very seldom is a plan put in place to help the patient deal with stress. Second, while you and the doctor are fighting the presumed culprit, valuable time is wasted that may affect your outcome. I heard the word stress in my own situation while struggling to obtain diagnosis for a rare disease the year before George began his cancer journey. Before his diagnosis, George heard it from one doctor also. I have heard other patients describe their first diagnosis in that fashion. If you are uncertain about the efficacy of your physician's conclusions, seek another opinion. We will discuss that issue later in this chapter.

You may have experienced a full-blown seizure with convulsions and loss of consciousness. For most people, a grand mal seizure with no previous history of seizure calls for seeing a neurologist immediately. This is not the time to deal with a doctor's office receptionist, trained to book appointments months in advance. A dramatic event such as grand mal seizure or automobile accident resulting from loss of consciousness should gain admittance to an emergency room with a neurologist on staff or on call.

Seizures are not always of the grand mal sort; some are quiet. A casual observer or person close to you may not notice a change in your behavior. There can be a loss of speech for a few minutes; the person might simply stare into space, oblivious of his surroundings; or there may be temporary loss of speech or a slight paralysis—just as when someone has a small stroke.

My husband experienced such a seizure. In a shopping mall parking lot, as we were getting out of the car, his whole right side suddenly became what he calls "numb and tingly." Unaware, I walked ahead to the store entrance; then, sensing that he was not right behind me, I looked back to see him shuffling slowly toward the store. He opened his mouth to speak and no words came. He now says that never before had he felt so frightened and helpless. He couldn't even form words in his mind. We have since learned that this phenomenon is called aphasia (loss of language). Within minutes, one side of his mouth had sagged. He looked and acted like a stroke victim. Fortunately, his power of speech and normal facial expression returned quickly. My fear of the unknown entity that seemed to be stalking our lives impelled me toward feeling relief rather than seeking answers for the cause of the episode.

George had little recollection of the temporary lapse of communication. If a person loses awareness of surroundings during a small seizure, there is generally no memory of what has gone on during those few minutes of blackout. Certainly, there is no recall of events during a grand mal. Therefore, a brain tumor may announce itself with grand mal seizure, a stroke look-alike, or a few minutes of semiconsciousness. These small seizures are generally referred to as "focal" or "partial" seizures. Immediately afterward, a person may remain fatigued and confused, especially if the episode resulted in complete loss of consciousness.

A sudden onset of double vision should be a signal to visit an ophthalmologist—an eye specialist. Double vision or any vision loss in one or both eyes also tells us to call upon the expertise of an ophthalmologist. Eye problems pushed George in the direction of seeing our regular eye doctor; ever since, we have thanked God for nudging us toward that decision.

Getting a Correct Diagnosis

Sometimes a patient is caught up in a series of events that result in bouncing from one specialist to another—none of them capable of solving the problem. You and your loved one or advocate need to be assertive when seeking a correct diagnosis. Stoicism, while admirable in many facets of life, is not a good thing when you are in pain or discomfort or when strange things appear to be happening to your body. The Brain Tumor Society has written in one of its publications, "The issue of delayed diagnosis or misdiagnosis is considerable and too significant to be ignored." One reason for delayed diagnosis is that many brain tumor symptoms correlate with symptoms from many other illnesses. If you suspect you have a brain tumor but have not seen a physician or achieved a valid diagnosis from any medical personnel you met with, study the list at the end of this chapter. Know your symptoms and check them off against this list.

If you realize that you have been experiencing two or more of the symptoms listed, make an appointment with a neurologist. Don't be distressed, however, if the initial examination shows nothing wrong. Persist with a second appointment one to three months later. Sometimes repeated examinations are necessary. Diagnosis is especially difficult in the case of children, because their behavioral changes can easily be confused with emotional and intellectual changes due to normal growth and development. Follow-up and persistence are essential for achieving a correct diagnosis.

Setting up an initial appointment when you suspect a brain tumor can be difficult for several reasons. For example, there is always the denial factor—as with my misplaced optimism when my husband displayed the beginning of aphasia (loss of language). Often it is a spouse or close family member who notices changes in a person's physical and intellectual abilities. This person may be the one who insists on follow-up, often against the protests of the patient. In other cases, you just don't know how to go about making an initial contact. Sara Gupta of the Brain Tumor Society says that many people have reported that their primary care physician or family doctor and his or her office staff have been helpful in setting up appointments and/or advocating for earlier appointments. Also, you can go to the Web site of the society (listed in the appendix) and look for the link "BTS Resources" for a listing of brain tumor centers.

The First Neurological Visit

Whether or not you have had a MRI before your first visit to a neurologist, you will undergo a basic neurological test, standard in almost all "neuro" appointments. There will be questions designed to test your cognitive abilities—questions such as what month or day it is or is the current president of our country. There will be an examination checking your reflexes, eye movement, sense of touch, tongue movement, and gag reflex. You will be asked to grimace and grin to show how your facial muscles are working.

Heel-to-toe walking will evaluate your sense of balance and coordination, as will touching your finger to your nose with eyes closed. As brain tumors sometimes distort the sense of smell, the doctor may have you identify various odors.

Technology in Diagnosing

Without the imaging techniques devised over the past two and half decades, we would not be enjoying the survival rates we experience in the twenty-first century. Two tests most commonly used are the MRI (magnetic resonance imaging) and the CAT (computer-aided tomography), sometimes called a CT scan or CAT scan. MRI uses radio waves and a strong magnetic field to produce clear and detailed pictures of internal organs.

When you undergo MRI, you need to remove metal jewelry and belt buckles because of the magnetic field. During the fifteen to forty-five minutes you are in the MRI machine, you will hear a loud banging sound. Some technicians provide patients with earplugs or music to help overcome this annoyance. Generally, having MRI involves being placed in a long cylinder for the duration of the test, but open MRIs are becoming increasingly available in certain locations. Check with the radiology lab when you schedule your appointment. Some folks may become claustrophobic—panic at being in a closed space for long periods. You need to discuss this issue with the technician before the test begins.

Your physician might order contrast used in your scans. The contrast material used for MRI scans is gadolinium, CT scans use material with an iodine base, so you might want to inform the radiology technician if you are allergic to iodine. Contrast is important because it concentrates more highly in diseased tissue, thus highlighting tumors. MRIs provide pictures from various planes, which permit doctors to examine pictures in three-dimensional images. I have known patients and their families to look at MRI scans, trying to interpret the latest results.

We still have George's original MRI—the one that sent shockwaves through the family. Someone had marked the tumor areas with circles to clarify the problem areas. Not all MRIs will be that easy to decipher, however. The radiologist report is the important tool, especially in the periodic scans ordered by your doctor as treatment progresses. Look for key phrases on the report such as "no apparent change." Since pronounced in remission, George's MRI reports continue to include that phrase.

Physicians need to learn as much as possible about the size and location of the brain tumor. To obtain a clear diagnosis, the doctor will order a CT scan to check for tumors in other parts of the body. If no tumors are found outside the brain, the patient has a primary brain tumor. If tumors are found elsewhere—such as in lungs, breasts, or colons—the diagnosis is metastatic brain tumor. The treatment plan for this type of brain tumor is different from the protocol (plan) for primary brain tumor.

So far, events may have occurred so fast that you, still in shock from the diagnosis, may feel rushed and out of control. You are entering a strange new world, one that you had never expected to experience. At this point, you need support from friends: prayers and assurances that they will stand by to help in whatever way they can. Do not try to go through this land of the unknown by yourself. Cancer cannot be fought in isolation. By the time my husband and I walked out of the consulting oncologist's office with the news of brain cancer, we knew we needed a neurosurgeon. We also knew that solid information on how to take the next step was a phone call away. The hard work was about to begin.

Getting a Second Opinion

You may wish to obtain a second opinion; it is your right and your responsibility. Most insurance companies cover this, and some even require it. A good physician will encourage you to seek another opinion. You will need a referral from your primary care physician, neurologist, or oncologist. He or she might even be able to provide the names of one or more second opinion doctors. When you go to your second opinion appointment, be sure to bring all your medical records, including your MRI and CT scans and pathology slides and reports if you have already had a biopsy.

If you don't know how to find a consulting physician for your second opinion, you can call the National Cancer Institute's Information Service at 1-800-CANCER for information on initiating the procedure. The institute has more than forty comprehensive cancer centers located nationwide, dedicated to outreach and education of the public, among other services. The American Brain Tumor Association also maintains a Physician Resource List of doctors available for consultation or second opinions. Call 1-800-886-2282. Think of your second opinion doctor as an unbiased observer who examines the facts that have been gathered. Second opinions are considered normal procedure among medical personnel in cancer care. In the past few years, pressure has been exerted on insurance companies to provide coverage for second opinions in cancer diagnoses.

Chapter 2
Preparing for Treatment

After long months of watching my husband endure a confusing mixture of mysterious symptoms, a final diagnosis was a mixed blessing for both of us. At last, we knew what the enemy was, but the battle ahead seemed insurmountable. Double vision had been plaguing George for several months, gradually worsening. An infection in one eye convinced us that we could no longer ignore the eye problems. Our regular eye doctor, an experienced and compassionate ophthalmologist, became our first angel when she conducted a thorough examination. At the end of a long morning she said, "George, I don't know what is wrong but something is pressing on your optic nerve. You need an MRI a soon as possible."

It took a bit of persuading, but the specialist currently treating George for thyroid problems ordered the MRI. When a doctor becomes frustrated with his inability to diagnose a disease that falls outside his area of training and expertise, he has two choices: call in a specialist for a consultation or forge ahead blindly. This doctor chose the latter; I suspect this was partly because he may not have known whom to call—and after all, he *was* the specialist.

Two days after the MRI, the telephone rang. It was the specialist. "Something shows on the slides. I want to see you in my office tomorrow morning." We arrived at the office the next day, protected by our naiveté—George's due to cognitive confusion and mine to denial. I wanted this to be over. I wanted a good ending. It was not to be.

Sometimes nature is kind and allows us to absorb bad news a small bit at a time. Many of us have heard the expression "God never give us more than we can handle," but I feel that many times He demonstrates more confidence in us than we deserve. The slides showed four large white "masses." I stared, uncomprehending for a few seconds, and I heard the word oncologist. "I've made an appointment for you upstairs with the clinic oncologist. He's waiting for you." The doctor stood up and moved toward the door, relieved, no doubt, to be rid of us.

In silence, we walked the long hall leading to oncology department. Entering that waiting room was like walking into a different world. Leaflets on cancer and advertisements for various medications lay in neat stacks on end tables. Soft lamplight bathed the room. A woman at the desk seemed to be waiting for us and greeted us by name.

The cancer specialist appeared self-assured and compassionate. After showing us into his office, he spoke quietly, telling us that the four large masses shown on the MRI were brain tumors. We needed to arrange for a biopsy to validate a cancer diagnosis. "I'll write a prescription for Decadron," he said. "It's a steroid that will help control the swelling in your brain for a while. But," he cautioned, "it's not a cure, just something to make you more comfortable." Then he left the room, closing the door gently behind him.

George and I sat, stunned and silent, looking at each other as memories of our forty-five-year marriage passed between us without a word. Then, I spoke as one stray tear trickled down my cheek. "Did he say brain cancer?"

We drove home in silence. Where do we begin? Who do we call? Friends and acquaintances in the medical profession are often good places to begin when searching for ideas and contacts. We entered the empty house and George headed for the telephone.

"We should call Kay. She'll know who we should see."

Kay was the sister of a close family friend; we had known her for years. She worked in the university hospital as a nurse administrator and knew most of the doctors in various departments. All the neurologists were out of town attending a conference, she informed us. Her next statement, however, reassured me. In their absence, the neurology department chairman was taking all emergency calls.

"Dr. Kindt is the best. He's been here for years. I'll talk to him and call you back."

By the end of the day, it was all set: we were to see him in his office the next day and bring along the MRI slides.

The initial diagnosis is only the beginning of a long and frightening cancer journey. You are getting ready for the battle of your life and this is the time to assemble all the tools you can think of. Involving others is one of those tools. This is the time to ask everyone you know for prayers and for whatever else you need, just as we did when procuring the right person for the diagnosis. You're not supposed to go through cancer by yourself. When we met Dr. Kindt, his reassuring manner calmed me somewhat, but by then George had lost most of his cognitive abilities and was beyond noticing much of what was happening around him.

I waited in silence while the doctor put the slides up on his lighted screen and examined each one. This office visit would determine what would happen to George—and to me—in the next few weeks. We had asked Kay to come into the office with us and I held her hand tightly, praying wordlessly, hoping that God was hearing my anguished and silent cries for deliverance from this nightmare. Finally, after what seemed hours, the doctor turned.

"It's not a metzi."

Kay's look of relief clarified my confusion over medical slang for metastatic tumor. I didn't realize at that moment that we were hearing the first bit of hopeful information.

Once outside and on the way to the car, Kay offered more hope. "I've never seen him call it wrong."

Dr. Kindt had been careful to explain the procedure for obtaining an explicit diagnosis: He would perform a stereotactic, or "closed," biopsy in the hospital. George would be given a mild sedative and a metal halo would be fastened to his skull with several screws. With the halo and a local anesthetic, his head would remain still so the surgeon could aim a biopsy needle directly into the tumors, using MRI images projected on a screen to guide him. This was May 2. We were to report to the hospital May 4.

Sometimes the situation calls for another kind of biopsy: a craniotomy or open biopsy, done under anesthesia. In this procedure, the surgeon cuts open a piece of skull and removes the tumor. The removal process is sometimes called a resection. When the detectable part of the tumor is removed, it is called a total resection. If the surgeon is unable to remove the entire tumor because doing so would damage brain tissue or because the location of the tumor prevents accessibility, the procedure is called a subtotal resection, sometimes known as debulking.

In diagnosing cancer, a surgeon might take a small sample of tumor, called a frozen section, and send it to the hospital lab for a preliminary examination, even while the patient is in the operating room. The process takes only a few minutes. For a more accurate, detailed biopsy, there will be a wait of about twenty-four hours for a pathology report on what is called a paraffin section. Treatment decisions are not based on frozen sections alone. Part of the pathology process is grading—determining the size and content of the tumor, a complicated process done by the neuropathologists.

Surgery is most effective for some benign and low-grade (non-aggressive) tumors. Brain surgery always carries a certain amount of risk. If normal tissue is destroyed, side effects may include impaired motor, sensory, memory, or visual functions. There will be some postoperative edema (swelling) even with the most complete removal of the tumor. In most cases the swelling subsides after a few days or weeks and can be controlled with the use of steroids, such as the Decadron prescribed by the oncologist we saw first.

I knew nothing of brain surgery or needle biopsies the morning I drove George to the hospital. A good friend had offered to go with us, and it did not take me long to accept the offer. I would need all the support and comfort I could find. All our children had been notified and were awaiting further news. The next hours would be focused on George and our future together. I tried to push away visions of a future without him.

I remember an overwhelming sense of responsibility as I drove along the interstate in a long and unfamiliar route into the city, hoping that I was taking the correct route. What if we got lost? No one could help me. All our married life, George had been the one to take charge when problems arose; he had been the one to take care of me. Now I was in charge of both our lives. I had never felt so alone.

Once at the hospital, I was allowed to stay with George and help him into a hospital gown. Something about changing from ordinary street clothes into hospital garb seems to remove an individual's identity. George looked helpless and vulnerable—childlike in his anxiety and unable to express himself in words. When it was time to install the metal halo in readiness for the needle biopsy, I stood outside the little curtained cubicle, feeling every turn of the screw going into George's skull. In moments, I felt a hand under my elbow and heard a voice: "Don't you want to sit down dear?" A figure in a light pink smock led me to a chair and placed a glass of water in my hand. Thank God for hospital volunteers.

Hospital waiting rooms have a unique ambience: a combination of despair, hope, exhaustion, and nervous energy. I entered the room full of nervous energy—the kind that makes one feel on the verge of vomiting. After pacing the floor for more than an hour, I sank, exhausted, into one of the large upholstered chairs. Would the waiting never end? After what seemed like an eternity, Dr. Kindt appeared, unsmiling and wearing his surgical garb—the green pajama-like clothing known as scrubs. He steered me to a chair in a quiet corner and talked softly.

"This is non-Hodgkin's lymphoma of the brain. It's primary, as I thought it would be, so we don't have to worry about metastasis." The words fell on me like rocks. I knew he was still talking, explaining, but I could no longer hear the words. They were disappearing in a thick mist. Then came one phrase: "Our pathologist is the best in the country." For some reason those words gave me hope—faith in the system we would be working within during the next several months.

As was shown on the MRI, and as Dr. Kindt explained, the tumors were deeply imbedded in the center of the brain. Surgery was not an option. I had to see George. I needed to see him without the halo. My friend who had been hovering nearby helped me to my feet, and we found our way to the neurology ward, where George was resting in a drug-induced haze.

In the days following his stereo tactic biopsy, George was confused: almost completely unable to speak or even to understand what others were saying. Worse, he drooled like a teething baby, something I had not noticed before the procedure. The medical staff in neurology assured me, however, that the worsening symptoms resulted from postoperative edema (swelling), a typical occurrence even with complete tumor removals. In most cases, I was told, the swelling subsides after a few days or weeks and can be controlled by continued use of steroids such as the Decadron prescribed by the first oncologist we saw. Doctors would keep George on Decadron, gradually decreasing the dosage throughout the rest of the summer.

One of the activities taking place behind the scenes while our family struggled to absorb information and deal with our raw emotions was tumor registry. Every brain tumor is reported, and the information goes to your state registry and is entered with other statistics on brain tumors. The Central Brain Tumor Registry of the United States (CBTRUS), a not-for-profit corporation founded in 1992, gathers and publishes data from individual patients' medical records. It receives information from state cancer registries, and patient confidentiality is strictly observed. The collected data is published and used in the research community. Copies of the detailed report are available to non-professionals as well as health-care professionals. See the appendix for information on obtaining a copy.

My world continued to fall to pieces, as thoughts and feelings tumbled about like popcorn. The man who had been my source of strength for most of my life was suddenly relying on me for everything from help in dressing himself to making life-changing decisions. I have heard other caregivers voice the same kinds of feelings, especially at the beginning of their cancer journeys. Receiving life-changing news, facing uncertainty, and gathering information on which to base life and death decisions—all while remaining a source of strength and knowledge for your loved one—is almost too much for one person. In chapters five, six, and seven, you will read of some coping mechanisms developed and utilized by caregivers in similar situations.

The day following the biopsy, doctors began final preparations for beginning the chemotherapy treatments. The plan called for receiving part of the drugs intravenously, so a PICC (peripherally inserted central catheter) was implanted in his arm. A PICC is a soft plastic tube placed in a vein. In George's case, it entered on the inside of his forearm and threaded into a large vein near the entrance to the heart. A few stitches secured the catheter to the skin. It would be my job at home to clean and disinfect the site of entry and to flush the line with sterile saline every other day. I should mention here that the very sight of blood or thought of veins—my own or anyone else's—has always had a deleterious effect on me. I have always been squeamish when it comes to medical matters. But one does what one has to do when circumstances dictate.

The PICC—sometimes referred to as a port—is used to deliver chemotherapy and to draw blood for the constant monitoring required to test the levels of chemotherapy left in a person's blood. George would have periodic intravenous treatments as a hospital patient and remain in the hospital each time until doctors were satisfied that tests showed his blood sufficiently free of toxins. We soon found that chemotherapy drugs accumulate in the body. The first infusion appeared to dispel all the stories we had heard and read about regarding sickness and fatigue, but as treatments progressed, hospital stays grew longer, and the drugs began to sap his strength and produce strange and ugly side effects.

Chemotherapy drugs would enter George's body a second way. To prepare, the surgeon drilled a small hole near George's forehead and inserted an Ommaya reservoir—a small neoprene cup. Attached to the cup was a tube the width of a piece of spaghetti, positioned precisely over the tumor area. Every two weeks we were to appear at the outpatient clinic, and Dr. Schultz would insert a needle through the reservoir and into the tubing, allowing the chemotherapy to go directly on to the tumors. This procedure is known in the medical community as intrathecal.

One learns many new words and terms when entering the world of cancer. I learned to write down everything I could about what was being done—the names of the drugs and any other information I was given. I found most of the medical professionals—Dr. Schultz, the fellow; Dr. Stabler, the attending physician; and the endless procession of interns and residents—patient and willing to answer questions. Also helpful were the information sheets the case manager or discharge nurse gave me each time a new drug or method was introduced. I still reread some of the sheets, marveling that we managed to survive those awful weeks.

A teaching hospital is not a very private place in which to be a patient, but the upside is the sharing of information that goes on within the larger medical community and the desire of staff to stay abreast of latest developments within each specialty. For example, while planning George's protocol (treatment plan or plan of care as it is sometimes called) one of the team consulted with the neuro-oncology department at Sloan Kettering in New York City. Sloan Kettering in turn faxed over a recently released report detailing survival rates of CNS lymphoma patients who had received whole-brain radiation (WBR). The results were alarming. The article, titled "Long Term Survival in Primary CNS Lymphoma," outlined a study on thirty-one patients with primary CNS lymphoma treated between 1986 and 1992 with methotrexate (MTX), cranial radiotherapy (RT), and high-dose cytarabine. Although the patients remained disease free, the literature listed some disturbing details regarding their recoveries.

The article continued, "Late treatment-related toxicity was observed in nearly one third of patients and those more than 60 years of age were at substantially higher risk." The conclusion stated that "combined modality therapy for PCNSL has improved survival, but relapse is common and late neurologic toxicity is a significant complication. Although this approach is highly effective for younger patients, efficacious but less neurotoxic regimens need to be developed for older patients."

Neurotoxicity, I have learned, is a medical term for irreparable cognitive damage. A paragraph in the report explained delayed neurotoxicity in detail. After radiation, the report stated, older patients in the study developed dementia, gait ataxia (stumbling walk), and urinary incontinence six to fifty-two months after diagnosis. Most of the patients eventually required custodial care. I refused to think of George's life deteriorating into such a state.

In other words, the report was telling the doctors not to use whole-brain radiation on sixty-four-year-old George. That was what Dr. Schultz was trying to tell us the day he gave me a copy of that report, as he gently laid out our options for the future. We have thanked God many times for the compassion and care we experienced from the time of diagnosis to the time four months later, when Dr. Schultz gave us the good news that the tumors were dead. The report that warned against whole-brain radiation was released in April 1998. George's tumors were discovered in May of that year.

The frustration from months of delays and misdiagnoses probably permitted us to enjoy the life we have today. George and I both reflect many times on our blessings. What if, we ask each other, he had been diagnosed two months sooner and had undergone radiation? All the time we had been praying for a diagnosis, God seemed to be withholding answers or solutions. The delay provided time needed for the doctors who would be treating him to gather key information. We have known for years that God's time and humankind's time do not always operate on the same clock; this life-saving delay proved another example of His care and protection.

George's recovery was not perfect, and our lives today are not perfect. There have been some cognitive changes: George has difficulty thinking of two things at the same time and becomes confused when faced with the necessity of multitasking. He needs more sleep. His short-term memory is unreliable, and he mislays things. But we accept the fact that we are living a miracle, as the doctors who have dealt with us are fond of saying. I like to think that to the medical community we are at the same time an enigma and a delight. We continue with post-cancer checkups at the same hospital where he was treated and attend monthly support group meetings at the same facility.

The Treatment Team

Most hospitals, particularly teaching hospitals such as the one we dealt with, maintain a formal hierarchy of staff. As mentioned, Dr. Schultz, who carried out much of the bedside contact with George, was a fellow—a person who has completed internship and then several years of residency. In post residency, a fellow undergoes additional training in a specialized field of medicine. A fellow in a teaching hospital works closely with the attending physician, the doctor who is the head of the medical team for a particular patient.

Dr. Stabler would be George's attending physician for the duration of his treatment; she still sees him twice a year for his routine post-cancer checkups. She is a hematologist-oncologist, which means that she specializes in both cancer and in diseases of the blood. George's brain tumors come under the category of lymphoma, which involves the lymphatic system—the tissues and organs that produce, store, and carry white blood cells that fight infections and other diseases.

The first year after treatments were finished, Dr. Stabler ordered an MRI done every three months, gradually increasing the time between brain scans until now they are done every two years or so. Unlike with other types of brain tumors that use MRI as a primary method for tracking progress, blood tests are also a tool for spotting recurrence in lymphomas.

I became acquainted with other hospital staff members that summer. Case managers maintain contact with doctors and assist with discharge instructions, making sure patients and caregivers know what medications to administer at home. He or she follows the progress of each patient and often goes on rounds with the medical team.

"Rounds" in a teaching hospital range from a system whereby doctors go from room to room, checking on each patient, to a formal hour-long teaching conferences attended by a large number of doctors and students from all specialties. This latter type of rounds is designed to benefit students more than patients. Watching the white-coated figures participating in the ritual of grand rounds is a memorable experience.

Nurses working in an oncology unit usually specialize in cancer care, including administering chemotherapy infusions for outpatients as well as hospital patients. George had all but the last four of his intravenous (IV) infusions as a hospital patient. Neuro-oncology nurses specialize in brain cancers.

Each time George was discharged from a hospital stay, the discharge nurse would provide detailed information on the medications he had received during his hospital stay. Even with written instructions on dispensing medications at home, I was plagued with feelings of inadequacy. I wanted to do everything right, and anxiety sapped a lot of my energy. Our grown children took turns flying in to offer support and help. I drew comfort from their presence, but I could see by their expressions that they also grieved and worried.

In some cases of newly diagnosed brain tumors, there is time to research and choose methods of treatment, treatment centers, and physicians. Our circumstances dictated more immediate decisions. George's gradual deterioration, occurring over the past eight or nine months, and his recent rapid descent physically and mentally did not allow the luxury of careful study. We were fortunate to make the right choices with the help of knowledgeable and compassionate professionals whom we now believe were shown to us by the help of God.

After George had been prepared to begin his first chemotherapy infusion, he was allowed to leave the hospital and spend one last night at home. As I drove away from the hospital with George safely buckled into his seat belt beside me, I had to resist a fleeting urge to keep driving until no one could find us. Once home, George sank into his favorite chair and lapsed into silence. I was not surprised.

An old friend we hadn't seen in a long time stopped by unexpectedly, in town on business. In the living room, I watched his expression change from shock to compassion as George struggled to communicate. After Jerry left, I forced a smile and turned to George. "Time for bed." Those last hours in our comfortable, familiar home should have been moments to savor, but we were too consumed with the next morning to get a good night's sleep.

Chapter 3
Definition of a Caregiver

As a caregiver, you are beginning one of the most difficult, frustrating, exhausting, and demanding jobs of your life. Becoming a caregiver is also one of the most important things you will ever do, whether you are caring for a spouse, sibling, parent, child, or friend. Caring for a person with a brain tumor carries a unique set of challenges. You are dealing with cancer and its debilitating effects on the body. You are also faced with the task of guiding your care receiver through a labyrinth of cognitive confusion.

Caregiving includes, but is not limited to, making sure medical bills and records are kept well organized, transporting or arranging for transportation to medical appointments and treatment sessions, and taking notes during those sessions. It is also helpful to keep a diary, recording you own feelings and thoughts during this time.

Involving Others

As with any type of crisis involving a family member, everyone in the family or household should be informed of what is going on with the person who has brain cancer. Denise Fleig, patient care manager at Advocate Lutheran General Children's Hospital in Chicago, says that it's a good idea to tell everyone all together and as soon as possible. In helping a family cope with brain cancer, you should acknowledge everyone's emotions, inform them of changes that will occur, and educate them on what will be needed.

This is especially important in the case of young children. Keeping your explanations simple and as free of negative emotion as possible will help children to maintain their sense of security. Family life and routines change in many ways during the fight with cancer. Some changes will remain forever. As the wife of one brain cancer survivor has said, "Now we have a new normal."

Early in the cancer journey, you should designate one person in the family (or in your circle of friends) to report the progress of your loved one. People want to stay informed, but you can't talk to everyone every day. Unless you are an extreme extrovert and talking to many people every day is an energizing activity, continually updating all those who are concerned will drain you emotionally and physically. Many people in crisis situations appoint a liaison, a person who will be kept informed on the latest news and pass the information on to others.

In our family of four grown children, all living with their families in the four corners of the United States, it was imperative that someone be the communicator. Using that method, I was able to make one phone call do the job of informing the whole family. You can adopt a similar system for friends and neighbors.

You are not going to be able to do this job without help, and if you're the sort of person who hesitates to ask others for help, now is the time to overcome your hesitancy.

People need direction in order to help, and they must be told what your needs are. Churches are traditionally supportive to members and their families during a crisis. I have talked with cancer survivors who confide that without the network of volunteers during the worst of their cancer journeys, they and their families could not have survived the ordeals as well as they did. Caregivers who ask for help are most successful in organizing a plan to preserve their own precious energy.

Know that when someone offers to help, that person needs to be assigned a specific task. If the offer is sincere, it is up to you to follow through with a direct request. You may need a prepared meal delivered to the house, or you could ask for help with laundry or childcare. Be gracious with your appreciation of the person's offer of help, and then describe your exact need. Look beyond the vague promise issued by someone to "let me know if there is anything I can do." That sentence is your cue to enlist that person in your volunteer army.

One man in our support group, faced with the daunting task of caring for his wife while working full time and keeping a household afloat, did not wait for friends and acquaintances to offer help. Instead, he stood before his entire church congregation, described his situation, presented a list of chores and timelines for doing them, and then instructed each person to sign up for some task, whether large or small. You may not wish to act quite as boldly, but that approach worked for him, and together with his conscripted army, the man kept his job while his wife took her treatments and the household stayed in some semblance of order.

If you need to look outside your circle of family, friends, neighbors, and acquaintances, you might consider looking into the services of one of the organizations dedicated to the support and survival of cancer patients. For example, the American Cancer Society can assist with arranging for transportation to treatment centers. You will find several resources of this kind listed in the appendix at the back of this book. Part of caregiving includes broadening your knowledge of available resources.

Finding the Time

Fortunately, I had no other demands on my time during that period of what we now refer to as the summer of cancer treatment. My part time teaching job at the college was winding up the spring semester just as George's symptoms peaked, and the last round of chemotherapy was administered during the first week of the fall semester. I was free to stay with him each day that he received care as a hospital patient. I also stayed with him when he was home, driving to medical appointments, running errands, participating in a support group, and indulging both of us in simple recreational outings that fed our souls.

However, not all caregivers have the same good fortune as I had with the blessings of free time during my loved one's cancer battle. If you are employed full time before brain cancer enters your life, you will probably need to ensure a steady income to cover normal household expenses and to pay the medical bills. One caregiver explained, "I kept working to maintain my sanity."

Much of George's treatment time was spent as a hospital patient, receiving infusions one day, followed by two to several days of blood tests to make sure the level of chemotherapy retention had lowered. Lengths of stay increased as the chemotherapy levels built up in his body. On one occasion, doctors kept him under observation for nine days. It was a very long nine days for me.

In the days that George was a hospital patient, I would leave the house after a quick breakfast and a walk around the block with the dog. Fighting rush-hour traffic, I would make the twenty-two-mile drive into the city, hoping to arrive in time for doctors' rounds. Timing my arrival was difficult, because some days the medical staff would begin the parade at one end of the unit and other days they would start at the other end of the unit. On a good day, I would arrive at the right moment to listen in on the question-and-answer session conducted by the physician in charge of clinical instruction. Often, the information gleaned from those events would spark questions of my own to jot down for further investigation.

The hospital days soon fell into a routine. The oncology unit included a pleasant lounge, offering visitors comfortable sofas with matching overstuffed chairs and ottoman, inviting weary caregivers and others to stretch out with a choice of the many books—paperback novels and nonfiction—from one of several shelves at the end of the room. There were informative books and pamphlets on various types of cancer, offered free so people could take them home for further study. Adjoining the lounge was a small kitchen where one could heat up a small snack. Most days I would bring a sandwich and store it in the refrigerator until lunchtime.

I could walk with George, rolling his IV pole, into the lounge to gaze at the large saltwater fish tank. Despite the circumstances, the ambience of the room was homey. Having all those books available provided me with a means of escape. Reluctant to leave George alone in his room for more than a few moments, I would read while he slept or watch television with him while he was awake. When he began to regain the use of language, we would chat quietly, with long periods of comfortable silence in between.

Maintaining Your Life and Sanity

Caregivers need an outlet—an activity or interest that does not include thoughts about medical matters, preferably an activity or hobby you enjoyed in the days before cancer entered your life. Hospital visits make it very difficult to get enough physical exercise; caregivers need a physical outlet to balance the emotional spending. For me it was the garden. Every evening at home I would putter in the garden—deadheading spent blossoms, trimming, weeding, and inspecting for insects. Gardening provided a great chance to unwind, to rest both mind and spirit. On the days when I stayed longer at the hospital, watching the sunset while driving home imparted a kind of peace as the sky turned from orange and blue to purple, then faded to a shade resembling one giant pearl.

Madeline L'Engle, in her classic *Two Part Invention: The Story of a Marriage,* tells how she would swim every morning before breakfast, reciting to herself verses of poetry and the Psalms, sustaining herself "by the deep rhythm of their faith" during the period when her husband lay in a hospital bed undergoing cancer treatment. I read that book before George's cancer diagnosis and once again afterward. The story held much more meaning afterward.

While caregivers need soothing experiences to feed the soul, don't be surprised if your emotions flare up occasionally and you lose control of the calm and controlled exterior you have tried so hard to maintain. You are in a state of grief, mourning the loss of a life as you've known it with your loved one and facing an uncertain future. Any emotion you feel is normal and you should allow yourself to acknowledge your moods.

Hysteria overtook me the day of George's first chemotherapy infusion. I had taken the day off from teaching classes at our local community college. That evening, when I stopped to pick up papers to take home and grade, I found a pink slip in my box, informing that pay for the two days I missed while staying at the hospital for George's first chemotherapy infusion would be deducted from the next check. I called a trusted friend who helped by listening to my ranting and venting. This was a case of the nurturer needing nurturing. I had not realized how close to edge I had slipped until that day.

You might sometimes feel your own identity slipping away as you become more deeply involved in the details of your loved one's survival. A caregiver in our support group once said, "I feel like I'm leading two lives: mine and his."

Caregiving for a brain tumor patient will test you in many ways. The person with the brain tumor may possess extraordinary optimism, may become depressed, or may exhibit bitter anger at you, the doctors, the treatments, and even God. All these moods may exist within one day. This is normal, and you must be prepared to deal with it. You need to maintain your own sense of self-worth and remain in charge of your own wellbeing. Taking care of your own mental and physical health is a part of caring for another person.

Early in our cancer journey, I received a copy of the Caregiver's Bill of Rights. This document declares that a caregiver has the right to take care of himself or herself; to seek help from others; to maintain facets of life that do not include the person being cared for; to be angry or depressed and to express negative feelings occasionally; to reject any attempt at manipulation on the part of the care receiver or others; to received consideration, affection, forgiveness, and acceptance; to take pride in accomplishments; to protect one's own individuality; and to expect and demand resources for supporting caregivers. You can add to this as your needs dictate. The full document is listed at the end of this book.

Your loved one might not need constant companionship or supervision, but if your caregiving duties require that you take time from your job, you might look into taking unpaid leave if finances permit. The Family Leave and Medical Act of 1993 requires employers to provide up to twelve weeks of unpaid, job-protected leave to eligible employees for certain family and medical reasons. Employees are eligible if they have worked at a covered employer with at least fifty employees for at least one year. The Hospice Net offers an easy to read explanation of the Family Leave and Medical Act at www.hospicenet.org. You can also contact your nearest Wage and Hour Division office, listed in your local telephone directory under U.S. Government, Department of Labor.

Some Practical Matters

Your loved one may have been the family breadwinner. He or she may have been responsible for paying the bills or keeping track of the many details involved in running a household. One of the most difficult and frustrating tasks of many caregivers is deciphering and keeping track of medical bills and records. Insurance companies can seem like uncaring, faceless, and hated entities at times of crisis. I have heard stories in our support group of battles and standoffs between caregivers and staff members of managed care organizations.

Keeping track of and paying medical bills at the appropriate time, and sending in an appropriate amount for co-payments, was the most trying task for me. I soon learned the importance of maintaining a complete file of medical bills, including dates for each procedure or office visit to be certain the billing matches the service. If you can enlist someone else for this daunting task, you will save yourself a lot of energy. I confess that I was a bit sloppy in my record keeping.

George had become a Medicare patient the year before, and we'd had little chance to test the workings of that particular brand of paperwork. If Medicare or some other agency is recent in your routine, you need to know what I learned the hard way. Your health provider bills Medicare or another agency, which in turn sends you a statement detailing what it has paid the provider. Finally, sometimes months after the service has been delivered to the patient, the provider sends a bill.

Before the hospital billing department had processed George's paperwork to admit him as a bona fide Medicare patient, it mailed the first bill to our home. The total was thousands of dollars. In my state of emotional disrepair, anxious to avoid a stack of bills piling up, I withdrew money from savings and paid the bill in full—at the hospital to avoid spending money on a stamp—no doubt startling the hospital cashier.

Fortunately, the hospital later refunded the portion of money covered by Medicare and our secondary policy. The lesson here is *do not rush to pay medical bills.* Let the insurance companies crank out their endless notices as they exchange messages with health-care providers. It seems like a waste of paper, but that's how the system works.

The system can also appear rigid at times. George's protocol called for a "rescue" drug, calcium leukovorin, administered in pill form directly after methotrexate infusion. This drug acts to stop the toxic effects of MX from going beyond killing cancer cells. Chemotherapy out of control in such cases would cause life-threatening toxicity to the bone marrow, mouth, and gastrointestinal tract. One day the insurance company and the doctor did not agree regarding the number of pills it would take to keep George from succumbing to chemotherapy side effects.

I had just checked George out of the hospital after eight days of blood tests finally revealed that he could be released and sent home. However, discharge orders called for a greater number of leukovorin doses than previously given. I watched as the hospital pharmacist argued over the phone with an insurance representative. After an hour of waiting, George looked ready to faint, and I had to get him home. I paid for the whole prescription out of pocket, praying that there would be enough in the account to cover the check. The bill came to well over $200. The prescription had been denied because it called for two pills more than the insurance company would allow. God bless the pharmacist; she pursued the matter, and months later a check arrived to cover all but the normal co-pay. By that time, I was too tired to be angry and frustrated, as I've seen so many caregivers become.

Many caregivers conduct extensive research on their loved one's particular tumor, available treatments, and brain cancer in general. A certain amount of knowledge is helpful in navigating this strange new world of medical terms, but there is a point where one can become overburdened. I have seen caregivers carry heavy briefcases stuffed with documents they have pulled off the Internet, and I'm troubled by the heavy load they are carrying, literally and figuratively. All you need is a small notebook for jotting down terms you need to understand and questions you want to ask. Don't hesitate to ask about procedures and words you don't understand. Most physicians understand when you ask to have something explained. Medical professionals have been steeped in "doctor-speak" for so long that it's a second language for them, and they sometimes forget that the rest of us are only beginning to learn.

Throughout the cancer journey, during the quiet times as well as the more dramatic, scary times, the most important part of caring for your loved one is just being present. It doesn't sound like much, but he or she depends on your being there. Love doesn't always require words or actions, but it does require your presence. Sitting quietly in the room, holding hands, chatting and reliving old memories, or simply sharing a companionable silence—these things all say, "I'm here. I love you. Don't worry."

Chapter 4
Keeping Your Loved One Safe and Comfortable

Brain cancer is like no other type of cancer. Brain cancer is a head injury, meaning you must care for a person whose physical, mental, and emotional strength has been assaulted. Your loved one's physical needs are relatively clear. Keeping track of and dispensing medications, as well as listening to and understanding what is said and done at each medical appointment and during treatment sessions are important parts of your job. The medical team will rely on you to carry out home care instructions and report any change or problem you feel might be significant. Two simple tools work best for this part of the job: a small pocket-size notebook and a pill organizer, preferably one with slots for various times of the day as well as days of the week.

Most medical professionals are tolerant of caregivers' non-medical knowledge and they understand our uncertainty. I found the nurses on the oncology unit amazing in their patience with me. One day I suffered a lapse of memory and missed giving George his midday at-home oral chemotherapy. In a panic, I called the floor nurse, certain that I had upset the whole protocol and set back George's recovery. No, she told me, he would be all right. Just give him the next dose at the usual time.

On another occasion, I again felt a pressing weight of responsibility when the discharge nurse surprised me with a packet of supplies to use when flushing George's peripheral intravenous catheter (PICC) and cleaning the insertion site. This activity was a first for me, and one I would not have freely chosen, but one does what one has to do. If you are squeamish about such matters, you must set aside that aspect of yourself and just do the job.

Diet: Meeting Problems, Finding Solutions

Knowing your loved one's dietary needs can be especially important when a part of the protocol dictates stringent guidelines. Procarbazine, typically administered in capsule form to battle lymphoma, is not compatible with foods containing tyramine. When the hospital dietician came to prepare us for the addition of procarbazine in George's chemotherapy cocktail, I was temporarily overwhelmed by the list of what I could not feed him. Tomatoes, pickles, most cheeses, yogurt, and bananas were only some of things I couldn't feed him. Procarbazine combined with foods containing tyramine can cause increased blood pressure. It seemed there were more items on the forbidden list than there were on the allowed list. Pondering the selection, I concluded that meal planning would be extremely difficult. Viewing my store of supplies at home, I experienced a moment of panic. As my husband's caregiver, I felt that his life was in my hands.

Sometimes the weight of responsibility blurs common sense. In a misguided effort to educate myself (quickly) on all aspects of caring for a person taking chemotherapy drugs, I picked up a book written by a woman who claimed to have saved her son from succumbing to a brain tumor by feeding him a macrobiotic diet—no meat or animal products. In short, the diet eliminated most forms of protein.

Dr. Stabler was adamant. He needs protein, she said firmly. He needs those building blocks to keep his body strong enough to fight the cancer and to ward off disease. Her advice to George was to eat whatever appealed as long as he stayed away from spicy foods or citrus, which would aggravate the membranes of his mouth and tongue, made tender by the poisonous chemotherapy drugs.

Everything I had read or heard told me that eating small amounts at frequent intervals is more beneficial than trying to force down large amounts at once sitting. Sometimes it helps to watch television or read while eating to take one's mind away from the idea of feeling sick. It is a strange quirk of nature that once we become ill after eating a certain food, we tend to develop an aversion to that food.

I served bland foods, and as it was summer, I didn't have to coax to convince George that sucking on popsicles would be a good thing. In addition to adding calories, the coolness was soothing to the inside of his mouth. I did have to sell him—daily—on the benefits of drinking plenty of water. The hospital staff wanted that chemotherapy flushed out of his system any way we could accomplish. The task became harder as the treatments continued. Chemotherapy has a cumulative effect. I have seen people who, like my husband, return from their first session of chemotherapy or radiation convinced that they would be able to sail through the whole protocol trouble free, only to find that they are not immune to nausea and hair loss.

My job as diet chief was made easier by George's craving for dairy products, ice cream in particular. Dr. Schultz approved of his choice. Don't worry about cholesterol or weight gain at this time, he advised. Ice cream is nutritious. To this day, one of our grandchildren asserts, "Ice cream saved my grandpa's life."

Dealing with Chemotherapy

We were fortunate to avoid much of the nausea that makes chemotherapy notorious. Only once, during the last few weeks of the protocol, did George's appetite completely shut down. In the hospital, the nurses and I tried in vain to convince him to take one bite of the soft diet dinner provided that afternoon. We ordered custard, but all my efforts resulted in George taking one reluctant swallow. Panic enveloped me as I imagined my husband slipping away in front of my eyes. That afternoon was a definite bump in the road in our cancer journey. There would be more.

In general, my husband tolerated chemotherapy well. Nausea from chemotherapy has earned a reputation as one of the ill effects, but drugs given before and during infusions help minimize nausea. When the intrathecals (infusions directly into the Ommaya reservoir) were given, he was offered Compazine, but after the first session, he didn't feel he needed anti-nausea medication. George experienced only one occurrence of vomiting during the entire summer.

Chemotherapy drugs are toxic substances; essentially, physicians are giving their patients poison. George and I have often reflected that doctors take their patients right up to heaven's gate, and then pull them back to life. We endured such an experience. About a third of the way through the protocol, the high doses of methotrexate and vincristine coming through the IV became toxic to George's gastrointestinal system. Fecal buildup and gastric distention became so painful that he later confessed he had asked the Lord to fix the problem or take him home. The gastroenterology department became involved, and a nasogastric tube was inserted. The whole event took place within a week, but it was extremely painful for George and scary for me. I was not in control of the situation, helpless to do more than stand by, watch him suffer, and pray for an answer to the problem.

One thing I could do to keep George comfortable and safe involved protecting him from the sun. Immediately after the first chemotherapy infusion, we visited our local discount store and purchased several large-brimmed hats. Each time he went outdoors, I made sure that he was protected with at least one layer of sun block (SPF 30 minimum) and one of his new hats. Think of chemotherapy as burning a person from the inside out. In such a situation, the skin becomes especially prone to sunburn; without protection, a dangerous burn can develop in minutes. The hat protects a head that has shed all its hair, leaving skin that has not previously been exposed to sun.

Chemotherapy also lowers the white blood cell and platelet count. White cells protect against infection, and platelets keep the blood from becoming so thin it will not clot, leaving a person at risk of bleeding to death. We were careful to avoid cuts or abrasions. Call me a bossy caregiver, but I did not allow my husband to handle sharp knives. To diminish the possibility of infection when going to public places, I carried a small packet of antibacterial wipes in my purse for the hands. Pushing a shopping cart, for example, exposes us to myriad germs that healthy people naturally resist. For people undergoing cancer treatment, the handle of a shopping cart, the railing on a staircase, or the handshake of another person can be a landmine of potential infection. Onlookers may have thought it odd when observing me wipe the handle of a shopping cart, but George did not catch any infections while undergoing treatment. I also practiced regular hand washing to avoid passing along possible infections in our home.

One possible type of infection, unavoidable in many cases, is a yeast infection in the mouth, sometimes referred to as thrush. This nasty condition reveals itself as a thick white coating on the tongue and, in some cases, sores inside the mouth. Alcohol-free mouthwash, baking soda mouthwash and toothpaste, or specially treated swabs will help relieve the discomfort caused by these sores. We used lemon swabs, bought at a pharmacy specializing in products associated with cancer treatment. We have heard of a patient who kept a supply of popsicles handy to suck on every time the burning feeling in his mouth became too troublesome.

Seizures

It will probably be up to you to provide or arrange for transportation to appointments and treatment sessions, setting up a network of volunteers to help with this task if you cannot be available each time. For some people with brain tumors, the responsibility of driving any vehicle becomes impossible; the threat of seizures, compromised eyesight, and skewed judgment due to edema (swelling) in the brain are some of the conditions that make driving for a brain tumor patient dangerous and illegal in most cases. When my husband was sick, I became the chauffeur to a man who had always prided himself on his driving skills and well-honed sense of direction. For months, he had neither driving skills nor sense of direction and was forced into unwilling dependence on me for transportation.

While seizures were not a problem for us beyond that initial episode before diagnosis, the subject comes up in support group meetings. Swelling within the brain can cause seizures, not only as initial symptoms but continuing throughout treatment and into recovery. Grand mal seizures are frightening to witness, but as caregiver, you should know a few simple rules. The fall 2004 issue of *Message Line,* a publication of the American

Brain Tumor Association, offers five tips in a comprehensive article on dealing with seizures. The society also provides these basic rules on a card to keep readily available:

1. Do not panic.

2. Make sure the person can breathe.

3. Clear the area of sharp objects.

4. Protect the person's head from being bumped, but do not attempt to restrain.

5. Do not put anything in the person's mouth.

6. Allow time for the person to rest and recover.

Another tip offered by another caregiver reminds us to place the person on his side in case of vomiting.

Immediately following a seizure, a person will be fatigued. There will be no memory of what has happened, and he or she may appear semiconscious. Remain calm and quiet. Seizures can be controlled to some extent by avoiding triggers: flashing lights, flickering shadows, and some action scenes in movies. Sometimes a person can feel when a seizure is about to occur. He or she may experience an aura. This may be a headache, a muscle twitch, a mood change, or a particular odor. Caregivers may become tuned into these subtle changes and develop an awareness that allows them to take their loved one to a quiet place to sit or lie down, making sure there is no gum or food in the mouth.

If your loved one has recurrent seizures, you should be in close touch with the doctor to achieve the best possible seizure control. This is most commonly done with drug therapy. Physicians often need to try more than one drug, or combination of drugs, monitoring the results to ascertain optimum dosage. The article warns that, as with many medications, people should not abruptly stop taking the drugs on their own. You can also contact the American Brain Tumor Association and ask for the ten-by-four-inch card called "Seizure First Aid." It's a good thing to keep handy.

Remaining Confident

The issue of keeping your loved one safe during the time you are gone will be your primary concern before you leave home every day with any degree of confidence. Solutions to the problem will vary, depending on individual cases. You may have a neighbor look in once or twice a day, or you may be able to come home for short periods during the day. Once again, you need to explore your community resources, including your church, your friends, and your neighbors. Some areas offer a program of respite care—volunteers who will come to your home and sit with your loved one while you take an hour or so free from responsibility.

Keeping your loved one safe and comfortable places you in a position of great responsibility. Do not hesitate to involve others in this enormous task.

Chapter 5
Challenges and Changes

Caring for a brain tumor patient will test you in many ways. In addition to addressing issues on diet, chemotherapy reactions, insurance companies, and medical bills, you are dealing with someone who has a unique type of brain injury. Tumors have pushed their way into an area of the brain and compromised or changed function of that particular area. My husband's tumors were located in a spot that controls language, among other activities. That would explain the aphasia he struggled with at the beginning of our cancer journey.

Your loved one's tumor or tumors may have appeared in the frontal lobe—the front portion of the brain that governs judgment and memory. Various moods will appear and disappear within a single day. This is normal and you must be prepared to deal with it, maintaining your own sense of worth in the process. Remember that you are not causing these mood swings. You have not done anything to provoke a bad mood.

The Use of Corticosteroids

One of the reasons for extreme and unpredictable mood changes is medication. I have heard caregivers share their experiences, and they match some of the challenges I faced when my husband was taking steroid medication immediately after diagnosis and during the weeks of treatment. I view corticosteroids as a double-edged sword: essential for certain medical situations but unpleasant in side effects.

The literature issued by the hospital on possible side effects for this drug lists puffy skin, swollen feet, headache, insomnia, reddened face, weight gain, muscle pain and weakness, and others. Not everyone will endure every side effect; reactions vary from one individual to another and in different degrees. Another occurrence I have seen in many people taking corticosteroids is increased appetite. My husband, having insomnia along with increased appetite, would enjoy a generous dish of ice cream at 3:00 a.m. many nights. Instead of the weight loss our family expected him to exhibit, he maintained his pre-cancer weight and even added a couple of extra pounds.

The purpose of the steroid medication dexamethasone, commonly prescribed as the brand name Decadron, is to decrease swelling in the brain. It works by preventing infection-fighting white blood cells from traveling to the area of swelling in the body, in this case the brain. Decreasing the swelling around the tumors eases the pressure of the tumor on nerve endings and relieves pain or other symptoms caused by the pressing tumor.

"Unusual moods" also appears on the list of possible Decadron side effects, a fact I feel the medical community does not sufficiently explain. These unusual moods can startle an unprepared caregiver when her loved one, previously amiable, becomes irritable, exhibiting flashes of anger or impatience. This unpredictability surprises a caregiver who already might feel emotionally stretched. If this phenomenon occurs in your situation, do not try to argue or reason with your loved one. I am not suggesting you should accept verbal abuse, but to maintain your composure, you may want to walk away. Say nothing and wait until serenity prevails again. I say this from my own experience and from listening to the experiences of other caregivers. One man, amazed at the reaction of his previously good-natured spouse, was heard to say, "That's not like her."

Be aware, also, that Decadron (or other medications like Decadron) is prescribed for short periods. It is not meant to be a long-term medication. However, withdrawal from any steroid drug must be gradual and done under the close supervision of the doctor.

An Emerging Alternative to Corticosteroids

An alternative to Decadron is being studied. Xercept, also known as human corticotrophin-releasing factor (hCRF), is a hormone found in the human brain and other parts of the body. The drug is a synthetic product identical to the hormone that occurs naturally in the body. As of 2006, the drug is in clinical trials conducted in various locations within sixteen states and seven Canadian provinces.

Creating a Support System

Coping with cancer is a project that should involve more than one caregiver. You are the main person, the link between the kind of life your loved one once knew and the struggle he or she is engaged in to regain it. However, you need company, and your loved one needs company. Socialization is an important part of healing and hope. If friends and acquaintances are reluctant to visit, you will need to encourage them.

I have seen people hang back from visiting because they don't know what to say or do. Assure them that nothing special would be required of them, just a simple hello and a five-minute chat. Cards and notes are special vehicles of caring as well. I have saved all the cards that we received because of how they made both of us feel loved. If the people in your lives don't understand how much your loved one needs their presence, it's up to you to bring them awareness.

Family members are also a vital part of the emotional support both you and your loved one needs. If the family, like many these days, is spread around various parts of the country, or even the world, everyone can still keep in touch through phone calls, e-mails, and perhaps a Web site set up especially for this period. Isolation is not a great healer. You need to keep it from settling into your cancer journey.

Celebrating Victory

To conqueror cancer, it helps to set goals. All through the time of treatment, I thought of the summer's experiences as one big project—saving my husband's life. George, on the other hand, was surviving one day at a time. I did not let myself dwell on the fact that months before we had planned a family reunion for our forty-fifth wedding anniversary in September. "Just a little more time, Lord," George would pray. "Just let me live long enough to be at that party." One week after George completed his treatment and MRI had shown the tumors had turned into necrotic (dead) tissue, we had the party. The following June we traveled to Hawaii, realizing another long-held dream.

Two months after our return we embarked on a cross-country trip, driving almost five thousand miles in three weeks, visiting family, exploring spots of interest, and stopping whenever we wished. We did the trip in stages, setting small goals and telling ourselves that we could turn back any time the trip became tiring. In the years since triumph over cancer, we still travel, although not quite as intensely. There are many more memories to be made.

Build Pleasant Memories

During that summer of treatment, we enjoyed some moments that have remained as pleasant memories, created during a time of distress and uncertainty. Whenever we found a small segment of time, and if George was feeling well enough, we planned something fun: small outings that would accommodate his lowered energy level and inability to walk long distances. Most people will go out of their way to provide what you need once they are aware of your situation. A local botanical garden conducted a private tour free of charge in one of their golf carts because we called ahead and explained our circumstances. The outing was an emotional outlet for George and a reassurance for both of us that handicapped people can be accommodated if only they ask for help.

We enjoyed our time at home also. Norman Cousins, in his 1979 chronicle *Anatomy of an Illness: Reflections on Healing and Regeneration,* tells of the importance of humor in the healing process. George was not able to focus his eyes on lines of print, and he was incapable of concentrating on the written word. The perfect mode of presentation for him was videotape.

We borrowed and bought some of the old classics: The Three Stooges, *The Honeymooners,* Charlie Chaplin movies, and others. The connection between humor and healing was explained later when I read Allen Klein's *The Healing Power of Humor.* Klein says that laughter opens us up to the world and helps us focus outward, expands our outlook, and gives us new ways to see our situation. Laughter, he says, helps us rise above our suffering.

Some television programs or videos brought sadness also. Moods changed often in those days. When the tumors were still present and the medication flowed through his body and brain, George would swing from happy to sad in a flash—laughing one minute, weeping without restraint the next moment. I learned to expect such mood changes. Now, years later, he does not remember that aspect of his fight with the disease.

The National Brain Tumor Foundation, in the summer 1999 issue of its quarterly publication *Search,* states that mood swings in brain tumor patients are rarely discussed by medical professionals, but emotional and personality changes occur in approximately half of all brain cancer patients. George's extreme mood swings gradually leveled out after the tumors died and new neuro pathways began replacing the disrupted pathways to the brain. At the time, however, watching his sudden emotional storms added to my feeling of helplessness and despair.

Music was a part of the healing process as well. We have always enjoyed music, but seldom had either of us taken the time to sit and do nothing but listen to a particular piece. That summer, any day that George was home, passersby would be treated to the sound of music issuing from our open door. I'll never forget the sight of him sitting on the garden bench, gazing at the brightly colored blossoms in my English garden and listening to the strains of Sandi Patti's rendition of "How Great Thou Art." Feeding the soul in that manner feeds the body as well.

One evening, toward the end of that summer, we walked around the block, George using a sturdy four-footed cane. His blood tests were finally beginning to show better results after infusions, and it looked as if his kidneys were no longer in danger. The gastric crisis had passed, and a recent MRI showed that the tumors were starting to shrink. When we stood for a time in front of our house, chatting with a neighbor, I experienced a feeling of liberation. How good it was to converse about everyday matters with ordinary people, not thinking or talking about illness.

Chapter 6
Support Groups
and Conferences

Support groups play an important role in the fight against cancer, and there are many kinds of groups to choose from. Some groups include all people touched by cancer, while others center on one specific type of cancer. People sometimes gather at hospital conference rooms, others at cancer centers. Some groups get together weekly, some monthly. There are daytime meetings and evening meetings to choose from. You can even find support groups online if outside venues are not convenient. Separate support groups for caregivers can also be found, dedicated to our special needs and issues.

Our Introduction to Support Group Meetings

Various support groups are organized in diverse ways and proceed differently during their sessions. My husband and I began attending the brain tumor support group at our university hospital while he was still in treatment. I noticed a flyer posted on the bulletin board while I was in the cancer clinic waiting for the doctor to administer George's biweekly infusion through the Ommaya reservoir. When I called the number listed, a voice crackling with energy came on the line. It was Bette, a woman whose husband had just undergone surgery to remove a Glioblastoma tumor. I would come to admire Bette and others like her in the following months for their strength and warmth. An extra meeting was planned for that month, she said, a potluck picnic in a park near the hospital.

The day of the picnic arrived and George was in the hospital, attached to the infusion pump. His blood levels were not yet acceptable for release, but he could have a pass to leave the hospital for several hours. Off we went, like two teenagers on a date.

"Goodbye. Have fun," called the nurse at the desk. "Be back by eight," said the nurse who unhooked the IV lines. Holding George tightly by the hand, clutching my little plastic bowl of potato salad and hiding behind a smile, I entered our first support group meeting.

Each group organizes its meeting times differently. The one we have attended for years meets at the hospital the first Wednesday of each month from 5:00 p.m. to 7:00 p.m., serving a light supper. The group facilitator introduces herself or himself and then asks everyone to say whatever they wish in introduction. Many people bring a caregiver along, sometimes a whole family, and all are welcome. During that first hour, we listen to a speaker or we simply share information. Sometimes we incorporate sharing with the speaker's program, as when the subject that evening was rebuilding memory, a huge obstacle to overcome when recovering from brain tumor. As a long-term cancer survivor, George offers encouragement and hope, especially to those attending for the first time.

The second part of the meeting time is reserved for caregivers. Along with a neuro oncology nurse or other professional staff, we retreat to a separate room where a tacit rule is observed: anything said in that room stays in strict confidence. The same rule holds true for the folks in the other room—the people with the brain tumors. This is the time for caregivers to vent anger, to confess helplessness or fear, to grieve for what has been lost and for what can be lost in the future. It is a time to say what cannot be said to our loved ones: *I'm scared of this thing that is taking you away.* Many caregivers are stretched to the breaking point, physically, mentally, and emotionally. A caregiver in one of the meetings expressed frustration over the complexity of dealing with insurance forms and medical bills at a time when his loved one needed him to spend time with her. It helps to know that others face the same kinds of challenges and endure the same kinds of pressures. Interacting with other caregivers dilutes the feelings of isolation, which can build to overwhelming levels.

That first encounter with others involved with brain tumors showed me that I had much to learn. Seeing people who had survived surgery and seizures and radiation and watching the easy camaraderie among people who had undergone experiences I could only imagine gave me the feeling of stepping into another world—a place I had been carried into, unwilling and unable to accept. I felt like an observer who had stumbled into a scene from a play in which I had not been assigned a role. I did not—could not—relate to these people. I wasn't like them, with their talk of BCNU and CHOP and radiation appointments. What did I know about those things when all I had learned was the word methotrexate?

The week following the potluck picnic, we attended the regular monthly meeting, held in one of the hospital meeting rooms. That evening would be our first chance to discover what goes on in a brain tumor support group meeting. At that time, the facilitator was Priscilla, the cancer center social worker and founder of the group. She asked each person to introduce himself or herself by name and by tumor type. During that period, I heard for the first time the word caregiver in conjunction with what I had been experiencing. I'd always thought of "caregiver" as someone with a job—a paid professional, not just an ordinary spouse or friend or relative. More than half the people in the room introduced themselves as caregivers.

I can't remember whether we had a speaker that first evening, but I recall listening during the second hour, when all caregivers moved to another room for our special portion of the meeting. At that time the facilitator of caregivers was Toby, psychologist on the hospital staff. Again, I experienced a feeling of looking on from a long distance, reduced to the status of a mute. The one or two occasions when I opened my mouth to speak, I was successful in producing only a kind of strangled croak. But one need not speak to be a part of the support group.

Years later, some of the group members revealed that when they saw George, pale and bloated, scalp laced with scars, his gait shuffling and uncertain, they were certain he wouldn't last long. However, everyone did their best to make us feel welcome. For my part, I felt overwhelmed and reassured at the same time. The brain tumor survivors and their caregivers in the group were going through much of what we had been experiencing.

Lymphoma of the brain, one person told me, is easy to treat. I clung to that statement for weeks afterward.

It took me a long time to gather the courage to speak at meetings, to share what I had learned from my experiences, and to express my ideas and feelings. In the caregiver portions of the meetings, I remained mute, frightened into submissive silence by the magnitude of what I was hearing, as if I were a separate person watching the scene from a long distance.

How Support Groups Help

Now I understand how the newly diagnosed people and their caregivers must feel when they venture for the first time into one of our meetings. George and I have earned the wisdom that comes from looking at death, and it has given us the ability to comfort and encourage others by offering advice learned from our experiences. Most of all, we listen because people need to tell their stories, as if putting the events into sentences enables them to gain some kind of control, to establish order in a world of disorder. By sharing our stories and listening to the stories of others, we gain opportunities for giving and receiving encouragement and hope.

In our support group, we learn that cancer is an equal opportunity disease; the importance of earthly possessions fades to nothing when people engaged in a battle against cancer come together. A person need not worry about personal appearances either. Radiation can do strange things to one's coiffure, and some people wear bald patches as battle scars. Some folks shave their whole heads and wear wigs, scarves, or hats, while others let the bald heads shine. A group of brain tumor survivors is a concentration of very brave people who defy an ugly disease.

Over the years, attrition and new patients create a fluid membership, but a kind of stability exists at the beginning of each meeting when we introduce ourselves and the word "survivor" is mentioned. When my husband mentions the date of his diagnosis, we observe the look on new members' faces as they quickly calculate the years of survival, then the relief that comes when they recognize a long-term survivor. We attend support group meetings to give back the support we received years before.

Over time, we have seen members of the group come and go, either to live new lives free of cancer or to a death perhaps made a bit easier for having experienced the kind of friendship and support that comes from traveling a difficult path together. Priscilla once said to a person newly admitted to home hospice care, "We've been happy to share your good times and now we are honored to share your bad time."

A comradeship exists among people touched by cancer that helps us come together to honor the life of someone we have known, whether for a few years or for a few months. We cannot ignore death, for in doing so we miss celebrating life. Living so close to death does not destroy hope. Everyone faces death, but for most people death is an event we prefer not to think about—something that will happen in a distant future. For people dealing with cancer death enhances the magic ingredient that hope gives to our lives: an appreciation of the moment. Invariably, George and I come away from each support group meeting feeling blessed and giving thanks for what joys we have had so far.

Each caregiver and loved one needs to search for and find his or her own support system—one that offers hope, comfort, compassion, and knowledge—all without what some would call a pity party. Support groups are far from being places where we go to find pity. Rather, they become a place to find strength and courage. My husband and I have been fortunate to find an appropriate support group without extensive searching.

Hard statistics on survival rates of those attending support groups versus those not belonging to support groups are hard to find, and support groups may not be for everyone. However, sharing your anxiety and sorrow with others can help ease stress. Lessened stress leads to faster and better healing for patients and caregivers alike. No one person knows all the tips and tricks of daily living under the strain of surviving brain cancer. Sharing knowledge is one very important way of sharing hope.

Finding a Support Group

Support groups for caregivers are springing up in various locations as the role of caregiver is recognized as vital in fighting cancer. For example, the

National Brain Tumor Foundation periodically offers caregiver training workshops at various locations around the country. You can find the latest listing on the foundation Web site or by calling the number listed in the appendix.

Organizations such as the National Cancer Institute or the American Cancer Society can help you find an appropriate group in your community. The NCI puts out a comprehensive fact sheet on support groups: how they help, who can participate, how to find groups, what types are available. Look for the fact sheet and links to get more information about support groups on the NCI site, listed in the appendix.

Brain Tumor Conferences

When the protocol is complete, or even between treatments, depending on how you feel, you and your caregiver might want to attend a conference sponsored by one of the brain tumor foundations or other entities dealing with cancer. For example, the large cancer center, M. D. Anderson in Houston, Texas, devotes a weekend to "Celebration of Life" for people touched by any kind of cancer. Each September, people come together to participate in Wellness Workshops and to learn about the latest research that continues to extend the lives of those diagnosed with cancer. Conferences provide a chance to socialize with others who have walked this hard road and triumphed. Banquets, music, and entertainment belie the grimness of this life-changing disease.

The first conference that George and I attended was a two-day affair called "Sharing Hope," presented by the American Brain Tumor Association. The ABTA, headquartered in Des Plaines, Illinois, presents many events each year in various parts of the country. The conferences, like many others, include a variety of vendors displaying information on clinical trials, research studies, and services offered by various cancer centers. In addition to enjoying the benefits of meeting and talking with other caregivers, I also appreciate the build-it-yourself ice cream sundae bar that ABTA offers at conferences. David Bailey, a longtime brain cancer survivor, is usually present at brain cancer conferences, entertaining weary survivors and their loved ones with his folk music.

We have attended a couple of conferences that included a display of hats donated by brain cancer survivors and their families. "Hidden under Our Hats" is an exhibit presented by the North American Brain Tumor Coalition and the Brain Tumor Action Network as part of many events planned annually for Brain Tumor Action Week, usually the first week of May. Throughout the year, the hat exhibit is displayed at various cancer centers, conferences, and fundraisers throughout the country. If you wish to donate a hat to become a permanent part of this traveling exhibit, look for the address in the appendix under Brain Tumor Action Network. You need to write your name, age at diagnosis, type of brain tumor, and month and year of diagnosis on the outside of the hat. If you are donating a hat in memory of someone, write the date of death as well.

Finding the Conference for You

You can find information about brain cancer conferences by visiting the Web sites listed in the appendix or by calling one of the cancer organizations, also listed in the appendix. Some events last as long as three or four days; others are mini-conferences of one day. These events are fine venues for learning about your type of cancer and for socializing with others. You might even feel pampered if the conference includes massages, ice cream sundaes, and entertainment. After weeks of grueling treatment, patients and caregivers deserve a little luxury.

Conferences usually take place in a hotel with easy access to an airport for people traveling from out of town. Registration and lodging costs are reasonable because hotels reserve a block of rooms at special rates for attendees. The fee to attend conference workshops and presentations is underwritten in part by sponsoring corporations, usually pharmaceuticals. One thing to watch for, however, is parking fees. We base our travel plans, whether to fly or drive, on hotel parking arrangements, looking for low-cost or no-cost parking. Many conferences offer one or two meals as part of the registration package, and some include a banquet with entertainment for a small extra charge.

Getting the Most from a Conference

If you will be traveling any distance to a conference, the trip itself can be part of a larger expedition. If time, energy, and cost constraints permit, you can treat yourself and loved ones to a mini-vacation, enjoying some of the area attractions. Some longer conferences are planned with sightseeing options for conference participants to choose from. Understand what you want and need from this time away from home. We traveled to our first conference excited to meet others and wanting to find more information about brain cancer, and we were not disappointed on either count.

Some degree of preparation is necessary to gain the most from any event; this includes using your time and energy effectively. Read the brochure carefully, choosing workshops that most suit your needs and interests. If two workshops that interest you the most occur at the same time, perhaps your caregiver or other trip companion could attend one and you could trade information and share handouts afterward. Try to take notes during the conference, or write down some of your impressions directly after the event. It's a good idea to take home information to peruse after returning home.

The most important consideration is your energy level. If you have trouble walking long distances, call ahead to inquire if a wheelchair could be available. If you want a room near the elevator, make that clear when you send in your hotel registration.

Above all, don't feel that you have to take part in every activity that is offered. Attending a conference should not evolve into an endurance test. Make your limitations known; it's difficult for people who have not experienced major health problems to comprehend some of the unseen disabilities of cancer survivors. Fatigue, one of a cancer survivor's biggest problems, is not easily discerned by a casual observer. My husband constantly hears comments such as "You look so good!" The confidence expressed by the speaker is at once reassuring and annoying to both of us.

Conferences held in a hotel usually provide a hospitality room, a place where attendees can drop in for a cup of coffee or some light refreshment and a catnap in a comfortable chair when the pace threatens to overwhelm.

Conferences are stimulating and inspiring, but they should not become exhausting.

I will never forget the first ABTA conference we attended the summer after George completed his treatment. A large white tent had been set up on the lawn overlooking a small lake. A soft breeze, the evening stars, and the sound of music lent a healing touch to my weary mind and body, and I felt all the strains of the past months melt away.

Chapter 7
Practical Issues

Meeting Lifestyle Changes and Challenges

Saving George's life became our summer project, with no chance to look back and very little incentive to look ahead. I lived in the moment, concentrating on accomplishing one small and uncomplicated task at a time. People deal with stress and uncertainty in various ways, according to each individual. For me, keeping control was paramount to maintaining my sanity. Staying in control meant keeping my surroundings in order. To stay busy was to avoid contemplating the future; there was no certain future to count on, and I had no courage to face the immediate possibility of becoming a widow.

During the days when George remained at home, gathering strength for his next outpatient intrathecal infusion or the next planned hospitalization, he watched television or listened to music. Reading was out of the question; he could barely process what was being said on television. The fatigue that comes with undergoing cancer treatment and from enduring the cancer itself is, to those of us who have not had cancer, unimaginable. People who have fought the disease have gone into a world the rest of us cannot enter. George's stamina diminished and all but left him entirely during his fight for survival.

During that time, I was left with the responsibility of running our financial affairs, keeping track of appointments, and learning how to make small household repairs. We were blessed, however, that cancer appeared in our lives at a later age than it has for others. Our hearts go out to those we have seen struggling with the need to be sure their families are provided for while incomes plummet and costs soar. Unlike in many families whom serious disease visits unexpectedly, we had no lost wages; our pension and Social Security payments continued unaffected.

Several years previously, we had been forced to adjust to reduced income due to a medical condition that dictated my husband's early retirement. We have often reflected that events preceding his diagnosis were a kind of dress rehearsal for coping with life-changing illness. By the time of our cancer battle, Medicare was the primary insurance carrier, and our secondary policy in effect at the time covered the considerable costs of chemotherapy and other medications.

Serious diseases bring lifestyle changes for everyone, however. George had been self-employed since leaving a large corporation. During our cancer battle, many loyal customers kept track of his progress, and we felt their support in the form of cards, notes, and calls. One customer even took us to his church for a healing service. For my part, dealing with new responsibilities introduced a lifestyle change, parts of which remain as a kind of legacy. Becoming a caregiver changed me forever; the future, while still uncertain, does not contain fear. I have survived an ordeal—walked through a fire of my own—and emerged with a new confidence that I can cope with whatever problem the future presents.

The lifestyle changes imposed on both of us during that period of diagnosis, treatment, and recuperation did not constitute permanent interruptions in our way of life. For that, we often comment to each other and to others that we count our blessings. Many brain cancer survivors, like George, are unable to continue working at the same pace as in their pretumor days, depending on the severity and effects of treatment and the residual damage done by the tumor.

Reentering the Workplace

After brain cancer, some people prepare themselves for different types of work, some continue their previous jobs with reduced hours, and some cannot work either during treatment or after treatments are completed. The demands of the job, the advice of the physician, and level of physical and mental endurance must be considered when determining future employment plans.

The National Brain Tumor Foundation publishes an excellent booklet, *Returning to Work: Strategies for Brain Tumor Patients.* The booklet lays out challenges and coping mechanisms involved in returning to the workplace. In determining your level of ability to maintain employment, it may be helpful to undergo neuropsychological testing, a series of tests conducted by a licensed neuropsychologist to assess your emotional state, and mental and behavioral abilities. The tests also help to identify the areas of the brain that have been affected by the tumor, giving a basis for what is needed in rehabilitation.

Multitasking is almost impossible for George now. He, like many other brain cancer survivors, cannot focus on more than one thing at a time and becomes confused when several tasks lie before him within a short period. The frustration for people who once were considered high achievers and high-energy people can lead to depression, so the key is to concentrate on strengthening and utilizing current abilities. There is a certain amount of grief to work through in this rehabilitation process, for the brain tumor survivor and loved ones as well.

Cognitive rehabilitation for brain tumor survivors includes work on memory skills plus as exercises to strengthen sight, speech, and movement, depending on which area or areas of the brain have been affected by the tumor and by the treatments. One thing not much discussed in the medical community until recently is something familiar to those whose lives have been touched by cancer: "chemo fog." One's thinking process can be slowed by chemotherapy drugs during treatment and for a time afterward. George experienced chemo fog, and we have spoken with others fighting various sorts of cancer whose thinking processes were slowed at least temporarily by chemotherapy drugs. Cognitive rehabilitation includes learning compensation techniques, which you will read about in a later chapter.

During one of our support group meetings, the issue of ongoing fatigue came up; it seems to be a universal concern among those who have battled brain tumors. The kind of fatigue present in brain damaged persons is a residual effect. Memory loss due to damage in certain areas of the brain demands greater effort in performing tasks involving thinking and reasoning. Most of us know from experience that a day of work involving mental effort is every bit as tiring as a day of doing physical work. Post–brain tumor life, therefore, may involve change in the way life is lived. In some people, change is more pronounced than in others.

When Steady Employment Is Not Possible

If tests and personal experience show that steady employment will not be possible, a brain tumor survivor can apply for Social Security Disability. If you are a caregiver guiding a loved one through this process, you need to know that the application should be filed as soon as possible, because lengthy waits can occur. Refusal on the first attempt is common. A first refusal is part of the routine in some states, and applicants need to reapply at once. Persistence is the key; don't become discouraged. For help filling out the forms, go to the hospital or cancer center social worker to get the process started.

We have heard stories of long waits for the first check. We've also heard of prompt payment. Be assured, however, that no matter how long the wait is for the first check, the amount will be retroactive to the date of approval—small comfort if financial life depends on Social Security disbursement. To begin the process of applying for Social Security, call 1-800-772-1213, Monday through Friday, to schedule an appointment in an office near your home. Be sure to ask which documents will be needed for the appointment (birth certificate, Social Security card, etc.).

According the Social Security Administration, "To qualify for disability from Social Security, you must have a physical or mental impairment that is expected to keep you from doing any 'substantial' work for at least a year. Or, you must have a condition that is expected to result in your death."

To qualify for SSA, an applicant over age thirty-one must have paid a minimum amount into the Social Security system during five of the ten years before becoming disabled. For someone under age thirty-one, this requirement is lower. Paying into the system means that a person must have worked in a job where Social Security taxes (FICA) were withheld from his or her paycheck, or as a self-employed person who paid self-employment taxes. The amount of the SSA check is based on past salary; the more money earned in the past, the larger amount of the check.

Supplemental Security Income (SSI) is a need-based program; an applicant is not required to have paid Social Security taxes. Someone disabled and with financial needs may be eligible if he or she meets the specific requirements for SSI. For information regarding requirements, call the Social Security office at 1-800-772-1213 for a copy of the pamphlet "A Desktop Guide to SSI Eligibility Requirements," or visit the Web site at www.ssa.gov. Unlike SSA, there is no waiting period for SSI, although it takes four months or longer for eligibility to be determined. Bear in mind that Social Security review files periodically. Benefits are retained depending on how a recipient might be able to function in the workplace. A neuropsychological exam might be called for even if the tests were given previously.

For those who have followed the application process and feel that they have been unfairly denied Social Security benefits, an attorney specializing in disability benefits may be helpful. Also, the National Organization of Social Security Claimants' Representatives is "committed to providing the highest quality representation and advocacy on behalf of persons seeking Social Security and Supplemental Income."

Look for the website and phone number in the appendix.

Medical Directives

Another matter for consideration is a medical directive—a document sometimes included in or attached to a will. The controversy revolving around the Terri Schiavo case, so prevalent in the news during the spring of 2005, raised a level of awareness throughout the nation regarding medical directives. If your loved one has not already created an advanced medical directive, now is the time to prepare a document that will be easy to understand yet comprehensive enough to be legally binding. When preparing the directive, there are choices: one can state that any type of life support should be avoided. On the other hand, a person can specify that heroic measures should be taken regardless of resulting quality of life. This directive may require some thought on everyone's part. Preparing that document, however, might save loved ones much uncertainty and anguish.

Five Wishes Booklet

In recent years, a booklet called *Five Wishes* has been published by Aging with Dignity, a nonprofit organization founded in 1996 and dedicated to providing families with practical information and legal tools to ensure their wishes will be respected. *Five Wishes* is part workbook and part reference book; it is recognized by health-care professionals in most states as a legal and binding document. If you live in one of the thirty-five states in which *Five Wishes* meets legal requirements, instructions in this document are legal and binding for health-care professionals. The booklet includes a card that can be laminated and carried in the wallet.

The document expresses:

1. Which person should make health-care decisions in case of mental or physical incapacity

2. The kind of medical treatment wanted or unwanted

3. How comfortable one wants to be

4. What loved ones should know

When people fill out and have notarized a *Five Wishes* booklet, they create a living will effective in thirty-five states. If one chooses to record end-of-life instructions with the help of a private attorney, the term living will might be confused with an advance medical directive or health-care directive, as described in the previous section. The titles are different, but they all do the same job: define what life-support treatment, if any, should be carried out.

As with documents prepared by private attorneys, copies of the sheets from your booklet can be made and distributed to family members and to the doctor. When admitted to a hospital or care center, a copy should be put into the medical file. *Five Wishes* booklets are available online or by telephone. Each booklet costs $5, or $1 each for orders of twenty-five or more. Look in the appendix for the Web site and phone number.

Medical Durable Power of Attorney

A medical durable power of attorney gives someone else the power to make decisions regarding your health care if you are terminally ill or badly injured. Another term for this job is health-care agent. This person can be a close friend, spouse, or other family member. The health-care agent must be at least eighteen years of age and in some states twenty-one years of age. This person should not be the health-care provider or an employee of the health-care provider.

Hospice

Sometimes, it becomes necessary to consider the need for hospice services—a tough topic and a hard decision that caregivers must recognize will be made by the patient himself or herself. For many people, the word "hospice" carries a connotation of despair and suffering. When my husband was newly diagnosed, someone brought up the subject of hospice and, without any knowledge of what that type of service offers, a picture came to mind of George lying on a narrow bed in a bare hospital room, waiting to die while our grieving family stood nearby, mute and helpless. Hospice is none of those things.

Hospice care is not about giving up hope, and it's not about leaving family and friends and moving to an institution. On the contrary, patients in home hospice care can become closer with family members than they would be if isolated in a clinical setting. Joanne Lynne, MD, director of the Washington Home Care Center for Palliative Care Studies in Washington, D.C., is quoted in the February 2005 issue of *AARP Magazine,* saying that many hospice patients find spiritual peace during their time in hospice care. The article, "Going Home," describes a man's final days in at-home hospice care and the effects on his family. One family member recalls that the experience was much more than a deathwatch. The man was cared for by family members and by hospice volunteers and professionals who offered pain-relieving medications, tucked soft blankets around his body to keep him warm, and massaged his legs and back to relieve tension. Someone was always available to chat or to sit quietly nearby.

Hospice enables loved ones to let go, recognizing dying as part of a natural process of life. When Sally Farrow of Arvada, Colorado, sat at her mother's bedside during the last days of a battle with non-Hodgkin's lymphoma, her mother was in hospice care at home surrounded by her children and pets.

Sally describes the dying process as similar to birth—both holy and beautiful.

Hospice care is relatively new in America, accredited in 1984 by the Joint Commission on Accreditation of Hospitals (JCAHO). Dr. Elizabeth Kubler-Ross and her 1969 book, *Death and Dying*, have figured prominently—along with others—in the early hospice movement. Kubler-Ross is credited with initiating change in the way the medical profession views the terminally ill; end-of-life care has advanced from an attitude of avoidance and denial to helping patients die with dignity and respect. Kubler-Ross identified the five psychological stages through which many terminally ill patients and their loved ones journey: denial, anger, bargaining, depression, and acceptance. Her plea for home care in the final days of life as opposed to hospitalization has made a difference in the way we view the end of physical life.

In the ensuing years, medical professionals, patients, and families have been able to work together to provide choices in end-of-life issues, treating death as a natural process, involving the whole family. Hospice programs include physicians, nurses, home health aides, social workers, spiritual-care coordinators, and bereavement coordinators. Volunteers provide companionship to patients and families, offer respite care, and provide help in a variety of ways that make life easier for families and loved ones. In addition to routine home care with hospice team members visiting regularly, a medical crisis calls for inpatient hospice care at one of the organization's facilities or around-the-clock care in the patient's home.

Patients may spend several months or weeks in home hospice care and then transfer to inpatient care the last several days of their lives. Bette Tunnell, whose husband died from a GBM brain tumor, says it was only when she could no longer care for him with home hospice that he was admitted to a hospice facility with around-the-clock attention for the last four days.

Tunnell has since become a hospice volunteer, working with staff, patients, and families. In addition to helping aides with routine patient care, she offers respite care for family members who need an hour or two away from their loved ones' bedsides during the final days.

Tunnell's most valuable contribution is her gift for talking with family members as one who has been on the same journey they are traveling. Hospice volunteers give of themselves, but at times the work can become emotionally exhausting. Bette remembers a time when two young men with brain tumors died within three months. "Things like that," she says, "are draining." But Tunnell and others like her continue to offer comfort to hurting people just as someone offered comfort at her dark time while her husband was in hospice.

Many people are unfamiliar with what hospice is and is not. Hospice emphasizes palliative care rather than curative treatment. The goal in hospice care is to make the patient as comfortable as possible when all aggressive efforts at cure have stopped. Hospice neither hastens nor postpones dying. Some people choose hospice care at home with equipment such as hospital beds and wheelchairs, and with medical professionals provided by the hospice center—usually a home health nurse and volunteers to provide caregiver respite. The prime goal is to keep patients as comfortable as possible and to live the very best they can with their illness.

If a patient's condition improves and the cancer seems to be in remission, either the patient can be discharged from hospice—home or inpatient—and return to aggressive therapy or simply to go on with daily life at home. If the discharged patient should later need to return to hospice care, Medicare and most private insurance companies will allow additional coverage for this purpose. Many people already on Medicare do not realize that hospice care is one of Medicare's benefits.

For Medicare beneficiaries to be eligible for hospice coverage, the patient's doctor and the hospice medical director must certify that the patient is terminally ill with a life expectancy of six months or less, if the disease runs its normal course. The patient chooses to receive hospice (palliative) care rather than curative treatment and he or she must choose a

Medicare-approved hospice program. Some hospice programs also accept Medicaid. The decision to enter a hospice is entirely up to the patient.

To find a hospice program, a caregiver needs to ask the physician or case manager for help with locating hospices in your area. Most physicians are familiar with the hospice concept and would be able to help start the search for an appropriate program. Your community might also offer information and referral services through the American Cancer Society. The National Hospice and Palliative Care Organization maintains a database of hospices for each state in the United States. The Web site is in the appendix.

Many people find it difficult to think of hospice and all that the term implies. However, learning as much as possible about what lies ahead and becoming familiar with the tools that may be needed to cope relieves part of the stress you and your caregiver and other loved ones undergo during the cancer journey.

Chapter 8
Angels and Hope

The turning point in our cancer journey occurred suddenly. Diagnosis had been hard won, with the primary care physician at a loss to find the cause of my husband's puzzling symptoms. The endocrinology specialist we'd been referred to was equally clueless, at one point suggesting that George try Prozac to conquer depression. Imagine the incongruity of such a comment against the discovery of brain cancer. When I learned of the presence of cancer, I was too stunned to be angry, but George fell into despair, thinking that a true diagnosis had come too late. He simmered in a stew of self-pity, angry with the first two doctors for their incompetence and arrogance. He was even angry with God for letting all bad things happen. "Victim mode" prevailed, the worst thing for someone beginning a cancer journey.

Then, George experienced something extraordinary. He had just regained some ability to communicate, to recognize that brain cancer was not about to take his life away immediately. As he described it later, he was lying in bed, consumed with fury, when a vision came to him in the form of a famous person who had recently died suddenly in an accident.

What are you complaining about, George? You at least have those twelve weeks to tell your family how much you love them. How much time do you think I had? You have a choice; you can be angry at the doctors who don't know of your anger and who can't change anything, or you can forgive them and reach out in love to your family and friends. Enjoy the time you have left, George, and let go of the anger.

Experiencing that vision was the turning point in George's attitude and in his goal to conquer cancer. He was ready to draw on inner resources to begin the fight. From that moment, he refused to think of anything negative. The focus from then on would be on the beauty of God's creation and of living and caring for others, one day at a time. The memory of that vision and what it told George continues to remind us both of the futility of anger. Anger breeds stress and stress feeds cancer. Love for life and love for others fosters rest and rest promotes healing.

Forgiveness, one of the many issues most of us struggle with, is an important component of the curative pattern. If George had not forgiven his doctors, the anger would have remained and festered, putting him under stress that would have interfered with his healing. When we gift others with forgiveness we also give to ourselves. Forgiveness provides a healing balm, for the soul. Richard Beckman, who practices and teaches intentional healing prayer, writes about forgiveness in *Praying for Forgiveness and Healing*, maintaining that forgiveness is the foundation for all healing.

It turned out that anger toward obtuse doctors would have been inappropriate in any case; just one month before George's diagnosis, a report was published in the *Journal of Clinical Oncology* regarding radiation therapy for brain tumor patients over the age of sixty. After pointing out that a study of CNS lymphoma patients conducted between 1986 and 1992 showed that older patients are especially vulnerable to delayed neurotoxicity after being treated with whole-brain radiation, the report concluded, "We now treat those over 60 years of age with chemotherapy alone, reserving radiation therapy (RT) for recurrent or progressive disease." Whole-brain radiation causes some amount of brain damage, more easily overcome in younger people, who retain the ability to grow new neuro pathways. Older people, however, do not possess the same resilience to overcome cognitive deficits.

The conclusion of the study showed that CNS lymphoma tumor recurrence and relapse is common. Delivering further bad news, the report warned that prognosis is poor for older patients treated with a "combined modality." Modality is another term for the method of employment for a therapeutic agent; in the case of brain cancer, the modality would be chemotherapy or radiotherapy (radiation). As described in chapter 2, this report on radiation was sent to George's treatment team in Denver just after he was diagnosed. If ever George and I begin to doubt the wisdom of letting God use his own timetable, we think back to the example of that study report.

Another important tool we would need for our cancer battle appeared when an ordinary person paid a visit, bringing to the hospital room a gift of hope. Charles was the first of many people whom we now think of as earthly angels sent by God to offer encouragement and hope. George had just completed his first chemotherapy infusion, and the infusion pump was pushing cleansing saline solution through his veins. Despite the fact that the treatment team had opted out of using radiation, we had no reason to hope for more than a few weeks of survival. We had been told that the treatments were merely buying time.

George was dozing in bed while I sat nearby. My thoughts spun inside a circle, never going beyond the safety of the immediate future. Within the next hour, I would walk to the elevator, descend to the main floor, walk down the hall past the chapel and into the busy delicatessen, purchase a cup of coffee, and return to the room to check on George. If he were awake, I would sit down and drink my coffee and eat my sandwich. If he still slept, I would slip around the corner and gaze at the fish tank in the lounge. That was as far as I could construct a future.

A soft knock at the half-open door brought me out of my reverie. It was Charles, a man from our church whom we knew only slightly. Our experiences had been limited to casual chatting over coffee after services. This day, as always, his manner projected calm confidence. Our conversation touched on everyday matters, and soon we were chatting comfortably like old friends. A half hour or so passed, and then Charles said, "You know, I have a cousin who had this kind of brain tumor seven years ago at the age you are now."

George and I exchanged looks. "How long did she live?" I asked.

"Oh, she's still alive. She's always loved traveling and she's on a tour in China right now or I'd have you talk to her."

When Charles left, the black cloud that had been hovering over our spirits left too. We both look back on our unexpected visitor that day as an angel who left us with a gift of hope. There would be more people and other events put before us in the following weeks whenever our spirits lagged and there seemed no reason for optimism. With an uncertain future, we gained courage from those incidents to face whatever lay before us. From the day of Charles' visit, we knew that God was with us and would help us every step of the way. A different kind of path lay before us—a journey of healing.

Sometimes the angels who appeared to reinforce our newly acquired hope were people we knew, and sometimes they were part of the medical staff. The hospital radiologist, while getting George ready for the mid-protocol MRI, offered encouragement, stating that his brother was a brain tumor survivor. Our retired pastor greeted us with a smile and a bit of cheerful conversation when we met him by chance in the grocery store. The manager of a popular botanical garden treated us to a private tour of the gardens. These people were all cancer survivors. All had walked through the fire and come out alive and strong in spirit.

Our grown children took turns traveling from their various parts of the country to make sure we were not alone. They came, they said, to help me care for their father, but in fact, they came to help us enjoy life. They drove us into the mountains, our favorite refuge in times of stress. They drove us to visit friends in nearby communities, and they spent hours chatting and looking through family photo albums. Our children and grandchildren nurtured us as if they were the parents and we were the children. It was comforting to have them with us.

Toward the end of the summer, someone made us aware of the R. A. Bloch Cancer Foundation and sent us a copy of *Fighting Cancer,* one of the free books produced by the Foundation. Richard Bloch, co-founder of H&R Block, Inc., was diagnosed with lung cancer in 1978 and given a life expectancy of three months. After two years, with no evidence of cancer in his body, Bloch and his wife, Annette, created the foundation, dedicated to helping other people diagnosed with cancer. In 1980, he began the Cancer Hotline, one of the first of its kind. The hotline matches newly diagnosed men and women to those who have survived the same type of cancer. Just as a hotline volunteer once offered hope to him, George now talks with other newly diagnosed people.

The second year following completion of treatment, George and I were invited to "A Celebration of Life," a cancer survivors' rally in Kansas City, Missouri. The foundation has built more than twenty Cancer Survivors' Parks in cities throughout the United States and Canada, part of a growing movement to promote a more optimistic view of cancer and its control. Each park is landscaped differently, according to the local climate, but all the parks symbolically recreate the experience of facing cancer and then celebrating the victory of survival, with emphasis on personal growth resulting from the struggle.

Visitors to a Cancer Survivors' Park move along the Positive Mental Attitude Path, which becomes more narrow and dark until it reaches the centerpiece of the park—the passage. Along the way are plagues, inscribed with inspirational and informational sayings. The selection that most impressed me was "Never give up. Never, ever give up." After walking the passage, travelers arrive at the triumphal arch—the highest point of the park—topped by an eternal fire. Passing through the arch symbolically represents seeing oneself in a different philosophical environment and understanding the predicament. From there, visitors journey down one of two ceremonial ramps that slowly descend to a grassy area. The final destination point is the Celebration Area, a small plaza featuring a bronze sculpture showing five people of various ages entering a series of doorways. The message one comes away with: "There is life after cancer."

The survivors' park in Kansas City is the first one constructed by the Bloch Foundation. Since 1990, Cancer Survivors' Rallies are held in the parks the first Sunday in June each year—National Cancer Survivors Day—with speeches, balloons, music, refreshments, information booths, and plenty of time to socialize. The rally and resulting media coverage help feed the spirit of those fighting cancer, and it demonstrates that it is possible to survive cancer and emerge from the experience with a quality of life. For those whose diagnosis has brought them to the edge of despair, the R. A. Bloch Foundation is a real angel on Earth.

In creating the foundation, Richard Bloch felt that one of the most important ingredients in fighting cancer is knowledge. "Knowledge Heals—Ignorance Destroys" is headlined in much of their literature. In line with the goal of creating the best quality of life possible to cancer survivors, the foundation has worked to get major medical institutions in every large city to offer a free multidisciplinary second opinion. Since the year 2000, more than 300 institutions at medical centers around the country have agreed to offer free multidisciplinary second opinions for those newly diagnosed with cancer. For information on this service and others, you can go to the Web site www.blochcancer.org or call 1-800-433-0464.

Richard Bloch died from heart failure on July 21, 2004, at age seventy-eight, having beat lung cancer in 1980 and colon cancer in the late 1980s. He left a valuable legacy of hope for survivors of all types of cancers.

During our cancer journey, it seemed that opportunities to enjoy the blessings of each day and to gain more reason for hope appeared with increasing regularity. The word hope and the concept that it carries appear every day in ways we had not noticed before brain cancer entered our lives. Maybe we have just become more aware of the role that hope plays in the human consciousness, and we're more adept at noticing signs of hope. From the lessons we have learned and the examples that we see in our daily lives, George and I have concluded that we all have an obligation to pass on the gift of hope and support each other in our cancer journeys.

Chapter 9
Prayer and Healing

Prayer and spirituality as viable components in healing are becoming recognized within the medical community as researchers study the influence of prayer on healing. Although results so far have been mixed in terms of pure data, proof of healing due to prayer, belief in God or another higher power, and their relation to healing continues to elicit the attention of physicians treating people with serious illness.

In 1988, cardiologist Randolf Byrd at San Francisco General Hospital conceived an experiment that he believes was inspired by God. The project involved joining Byrd's two deepest commitments: science and faith. Over a ten-month period, 393 patients in the hospital coronary care unit agreed to participate in either a group that would be prayed for or a group that would receive no prayer at all. As with all good clinical experiments, randomization and double blind precautions were employed. Neither patients nor their doctors and nurses knew who was being prayed for and who was not receiving prayer.

Dr. Byrd recruited members of several Protestant and Roman Catholic groups from around the country to pray. Other than patients' first names and medical conditions, the volunteers were given no instructions other than to pray each day. Each of the patients in the group being prayed for had five to seven people praying for him or her. The results of the study were startling. The overall rate of complications and mortality was much lower in the prayed-for group than in the group whose members had received no prayer.

Dr. Larry Dossey is another physician who looks at prayer as a healing tool. "Prayer," says Dossey, "is good medicine." The basis of prayer is the creation of hope. Hope heals, he says, and hopelessness kills. To avoid the false expectation that someone being prayed for will suddenly recover one hundred percent, Dossey cites a spectrum of hope. At one end is an unrealistic expectation of healing, while at the other there is a "doomsday" prediction. Unrealistic expectations convey false notions of what recovery is. Recovery from any kind of serious illness does not imply that a person is physically or emotionally the same as before the illness. A doomsday prediction implies that serious illness will result in immediate death. We need to stand somewhere in the middle, where the dominant factor is love.

Although the split between religion and science is narrowing, the idea of prayer and healing is not without critics. Since Byrd's original study, more studies have been done and more critics have stepped up with the same argument that hard, quantified data is impossible to obtain. Critics of Byrd's study on prayer argue that it is difficult to accurately study effects of prayer on critically ill patients, pointing out that in dire circumstances, people pray for themselves and their loved ones pray for them as well, making it impossible to establish a pure control group.

Carrying further the notion of intercessional prayer, Dossey points to examples of people praying for nonhuman subjects—veterinarians praying for their patients, farmers praying for their plants and animals—with positive results overall. He feels that it is impossible to overcome all major resistances to prayer research by doing experiments in non-humans. When prayer for critically ill people fails to result in complete healing, skeptics of healing prayer could claim that prayer creates false hope. Dossey counters by comparing healing with therapy. All medicines, he says, have a failure rate. As with therapy, sometimes prayer works and sometimes it does not. We cannot know in advance, what the outcome will be. But, says Dossey, if he were seriously ill, he would try to get on as many prayer lists as possible while undergoing medical treatment. As long as studies show positive effects, he concludes, why not try prayer?

We may never obtain enough facts to determine the efficacy of prayer in healing. Faith healing and healing through prayer carry different connotations. Many of us have viewed or heard about severely disabled people rising from their wheelchairs and walking unaided for the first time in years. The studies being done on prayer and healing do not document such phenomena. Dr. Mitchell W. Krucoff of Duke University concedes that a person's point of view shades the individual interpretation of these studies. However, he and others agree that it is important to study prayer as an adjunct—not a replacement—to standard medical care.

In 2002, Dr. Ed Arenson, a neuro-oncologist at one of Denver's leading hospitals, began holding monthly interfaith spiritual healing services for cancer patients and their loved ones because, he says, "patients have needs that extend beyond physical needs." Arenson conceived the idea of a spiritual service from a similar service he attended at synagogue. Many of the readings, prayers, and melodies are rooted in the Hebrew tradition and modified to appeal to the broader, predominately non-Jewish groups who attend the services.

Patients, family, and hospital staff gather once a month to participate in meditative hymns and chants, praying both silently and aloud. The gatherings are organized by the Colorado Neurological Institute for Brain and Spinal Tumors in conjunction with the chaplain's office at Swedish Hospital in Englewood, Colorado. Spiritual comfort is also extended to caregivers, and periodic meetings are held for those whose loved ones have lost their cancer battles.

Prayer and hope join in tying faith and science. Oncologist-hematologist Dr. Jerome Groopman in his book *Anatomy of Hope: How People Prevail in the Face of Illness* describes a colleague diagnosed with advanced cancer and his struggle to reconcile science and religion. The patient drew great comfort from intercessional prayers put forth by fellow scientists of many faiths: Christians, Jews, Hindus, Buddhists, and Muslims. As he became hopeful of surviving, he was cured of cancer. Groopman believes that the main ingredient in faith is hope. With hope comes a sense of control and a feeling of peace—of being able to accept whatever will occur. Hope turns off the negative emotions that create fear and depression. Groopman believes that in using hope to lessen fear, we can recognize the dangers in a grave situation, thereby relieving anxiety and giving us strength to endure.

When God's notion of healing does not necessarily involve continuing one's life on Earth, healing can mean a peaceful death of the body. Acceptance of one's situation heals the spirit and lessens the pain of those left behind. Through the years, George and I have seen people who have prayed for death after a period of suffering. We once took part in a healing, with a laying on of hands, for a friend with lung cancer that had metastasized to the brain, rendering the person angry and despairing. Our prayer was for peace of spirit and reconciliation, not absolute healing of the body. We knew that God was ultimately in charge of the situation and that we were only instruments. We will never know exactly why some people live through horrifying ordeals and others do not. The gift of survival is often laced with unanswered questions. We have concluded that the best way to cope with survival is to honor the gift of life by passing on hope—in all of its embodiments—to others.

When George's body began to fail him in the spring of 1998 and no one could tell us the cause, he called our pastor and together they prayed for a valid diagnosis. Within a week, a routine visit to our ophthalmologist for treatment of an eye infection put in motion events leading the discovery of the tumors in his brain. God did not make those tumors disappear the day the MRI was done, nor did the tumors go away immediately after the diagnosis or even after treatment began. God, however, did lead us gradually through the things we needed to do. He kept us strengthened to get through each day, and he guided the medical personnel in charge of George's care. We were prayed for. Some prayers we knew of and some we may never know about.

After treatment was completed and George's thinking capacities began to return, he prayed for the ability to communicate the story of his triumph over cancer. He wanted to share his joy with our children and grandchildren. In one afternoon, he wrote several pages conveying his feelings and blessing from God. On one of those pages, George compared his situation to that of Job in the Bible, when Satan took away all of Job's possessions and his good health. Job never lost faith in God. Ultimately God gave back to Job twice what was lost to Satan. George now says that he feels blessed that he had brain cancer; it helped to put his life in perspective, with time left to set new priorities and share thoughts with family and friends, testing new ways of praying for knowledge, strength, inspiration, and patience for things to happen in God's time, not ours.

Besides George's own prayers and the prayers of others, we experienced two healing services. One was held in a church as part of a larger service. The second event took place in our home with a friend and two other women from her church. The home service was different from anything I had experienced in the past. As George and I had not previously met the two women who arrived with my friend, there was a period of getting acquainted, chatting about ordinary things, and building an atmosphere of trust among the five of us. My feeling was, and still is, that in order for a healing to work as it should, one must have perfect trust in the healer. The healer is the hands and heart of God, his tools.

After about an hour of conversation, one of the women asked George what kind of healing he would ask for. Did he want the tumors to go away completely, never to return, or did he just want some extra time? I waited for what seemed minutes before the answer came. He had already asked God for a few extra weeks beyond what the doctors had predicted. What would he say now?

"I think I want the tumors to go away."

We began. George sat in his favorite chair, looking relaxed and expectant, while the rest of us gathered around him to place our hands on his shoulders and head. Sally and Cloetta prayed aloud, calling upon the healing powers of God to remove the cancer from George's body. Sally had brought a vial of oil, and she put a few drops on her thumb to make the sign of the cross on George's forehead. With my hand on George's shoulder, I willed my energy to pass from my body into his as I prayed that life from my spirit would flow through me and into George. He later said that during the prayers he felt warmth go through his entire body and settle on him like a soft, comforting blanket.

That afternoon, George did not leap from his chair, instantly and miraculously healed as is seen on some televised healers' services. Instead, he felt a deep inner peace that exceeds human understanding. Having participated in the laying on of hands, I felt the same kind of peace. Looking back, I know it was God revealing himself to us in his own quiet, mysterious way. Years later, Sally confided that George's openness to whatever might happen made him a perfect candidate for healing.

People who have the gift of healing can tell us that there are many forms of healing. Some physical healing is gradual, as in George's case. Weeks after the home healing service, a routine mid-protocol MRI showed the tumors had shrunk to half their original size. It was not until the last infusion had been completed that another MRI showed that all four tumors had died. All that remained was necrosis (dead tissue) where live and growing tumors once had been. Some healings are sudden, although they happen quietly. Stories are told of people with malignant tumors that disappear as though by magic. I cannot dispute those stories, only accept them as part of God's ways.

Some people, I was later told, cling to a disease, and after a while it becomes part of their identity, becoming "my cancer." We have learned never to speak of cancer as "my cancer" or "his cancer." Cancer is an unwelcome presence in your body and it is your job to make it feel as alien and unwanted as you possibly can. I remember attending a brain tumor conference where a man in his thirtieth year of surviving a glioblastoma multiforme spoke of standing in front of a mirror each day. In a loud voice, he would order the cancer cells to go away. *Thirty years!* My thought at that moment was, "Whatever works." George used to imagine little Pac-men chewing away at the cells. One woman told me that she visualized angels flying away with cancer cells.

George's inner peace and faith in God kept him fast in the belief that he was in a win-win situation. He would either become free of cancer or he would go to heaven; it was for God to make the ultimate decision. Sometimes people who have prayed, and have been prayed for, die anyway. There can remain for those left behind a sense of abandonment and failure, the feeling that no one prayed hard enough or well enough. Our God is not a vengeful God, and we do not have to live up to a certain standard of behavior or practice a particular quality of prayer. Just as the medical doctors tell us there is no apparent reason for brain cancer, there also is no obvious reason for who survives and who does not. There is no answer to the question that George asks: Why not me? Why did I survive when others do not? Why did he survive against all odds? We may never know.

A particular television program caught George's interest after he finished his treatments and began the process of adapting to survival. Bill Moyers' public television series *Healing and the Mind* illustrates the importance of physicians going beyond practicing the mechanics of medicine and taking the role of healers. Medical professionals are starting to recognize the importance of instilling and nurturing hope in their patients, for when hope is gone life soon dies. I have heard of doctors who believe in telling the truth to people whose cancer is far advanced. These doctors in their earnest efforts to avoid giving false hope when all their training indicates that there is no hope can either impart a sense of despair or inspire a person to fight harder. Unfortunately, the latter is less common than the former.

George and I often think of Dr. Schultz and his gentle way of presenting the options for treating George's brain cancer. In the end, the choice would be ours, and we chose the aggressive protocol—the course of action that was expected only to prolong life by a few weeks. As we signed the papers to begin the treatments, Dr. Schultz assured us that his prayers would be with us throughout the protocol. We were fortunate to have a doctor whose belief in prayer was a part of his practice when treating disease.

After George survived the whole course of treatment, we were told that he might not live out the year. We did a lot of celebrating in that year, fitting in as much fun and joy of living as possible, at the same time denying and defying the expectations of the medical professionals. Doctors now look at him and say, "George, you are a miracle."

Scientific research on predicting, diagnosing, and treating brain tumors continues. Clinical trials and studies continue to produce new methods of delivery and new medications to battle brain cancer, but in the end, good medical practice means more than fixing bodies with scientific techniques.

Chapter 10
The Job of Survival

After a person has been declared cancer free, there may be a mix of emotions. In our case, news of the tumors' demise was communicated to us over the telephone. Four short words: "The tumors are dead." Dr. Schultz had to repeat the sentence three times before my mind absorbed the good news. If he had been standing in front of us, I would have hugged him. George, who had been listening on the other line, sounded equally baffled. After we hung up the phone, we stared at each other, speechless. Then, filled with elation, we wanted to tell the whole world. We hadn't been so jubilant since our first grandchild was born.

Then, as I suspect in many cases, reality settled in and we were left with the task of constructing a new life—finding what many brain tumor survivors refer to as a "new normal." After weeks or months of putting one's life on hold, focusing only on surviving day by day, making long-term commitments and setting goals does not come easily. When we first hear of remission of a life-stealing disease, the human spirit may soar in joy, but it must also return to Earth to face daily living. We needed to figure out what to do next.

First, we celebrated. We hosted a party at a mountain resort where George and I renewed our wedding vows under a stately pine tree in the presence of friends and family. Everyone toasted our forty-fifth anniversary and there was food and music and lively conversation laced with hearty laughter. It was glorious. A young female deer even came to the party, walking with dainty footsteps among a group of people standing outside. George was still somewhat confused and very fatigued, but he was alive and that was all I wanted to concentrate on at that time.

When survivors are pronounced in remission, they have earned it, just as a runner winning a race deserves the medal. However, after the euphoria has subsided and they have absorbed the good news, patient and caregiver both will need support, just as they needed support during the long ordeal of treatments. Support groups exist for survivors just as they offer care and comfort for those still in the battle.

Support groups can be an important way of easing into post-cancer life. The groups usually include other people dealing with issues of rebuilding lives after brain cancer. Newcomers to a brain tumor support group need to see survivors—those who have been pronounced in remission. George and I continue to attend monthly brain tumor support group meetings to offer support just as we gained support years ago. Newly diagnosed people and their loved ones need to meet and talk with seasoned veterans who give the message *we made it through and you can too.* Observing others survive a cancer journey that they themselves are just beginning inspires and encourages. It is difficult to correlate survival with support group attendance, but I have learned of many caregivers and loved ones who say that being in a support group has given them courage and hope.

Survivors have many chances to pass on to others what they have learned from experience. In addition to attending support group meetings, there are opportunities to volunteer in other ways. Churches, cancer center hotlines, and hospice facilities all provide the kind of support and information for which many people beginning a cancer journey hunger. Just after our celebration party, George put his name on the Richard Bloch Cancer Hotline volunteer list. He receives calls from the hotline and speaks with people battling various types of brain tumors as well as non-Hodgkin's lymphoma.

Sometimes I am called upon to speak with another caregiver. Frequently, George is unable to answer questions about his protocol or events that transpired while he was particularly confused. Then, I am summoned to the telephone. Often a person is depressed, discouraged because of lingering fatigue. One such person pressed me to offer a date when she might expect to regain her strength. In dealing with a difficult question such as this one, I try to remain neutral, not discouraging but not dismissive. One person's pain and fatigue may be an overpowering burden, whereas, to another person, pain or loss of energy is only a slight inconvenience. Everyone is different. However, there is always something to celebrate: the gift of life, whether for one year, many years, or one day.

Hotline volunteers are free to explain in lay terms what they experienced during treatment and describe how various drugs affected them, cautioning that what might work for one person might not work for another. Volunteers are the perfect candidates to offer tips on getting through treatments and side effects, based on what they found helpful for themselves. For the callers, fear of the unknown can be erased, clearing the path for treatments to work effectively.

Hotline volunteers are also free to recommend the benefits of second opinions during the first step in someone's cancer journey in order to make informed, correct decisions. Circumstances surrounding George's onset of symptoms dictated haste. Many people, however, can and should take the time to make informed, deliberate choices regarding their treatment plans. Lay people in volunteer roles need to refrain from offering medical advice. The job of volunteers is to offer hope through sharing good news. George and I once visited a man whose caregiver stood by his bedside, distraught and despairing until we mentioned the cancer hotline. You can speak with other survivors, we told her. At the word *survivor*, a visible change came over both the man and his wife; their faces brightened as if a cloud had lifted. They had hope.

Just after our official remission pronouncement, George and I vacillated between relief and wariness. We were relieved that the tumors were dead. We were also terrified that either there had been a mistake and the tumors were still viable or that the tumors would return soon, as doctors had warned. Then, a CNS lymphoma survivor called from the hotline at M. D. Anderson, the large cancer center in Houston, Texas. I couldn't believe my ears: someone who had lived for five years in remission. That news came at a time when George's physicians were cautioning him to get his affairs in order within the year, because CNS lymphoma always comes back. We owe a debt of gratitude to Bobby Blum for offering that gift of hope in the form of live proof that survival can be long term.

Over the years, friends, neighbors, family members have called on George to speak with someone newly diagnosed with brain cancer. Sometimes a caregiver wants to talk to me. We accept the challenge, gratefully and humbly. It is a chance to give back what was given to us.

Brain tumor conferences and cancer survivor celebrations present great opportunities to offer hope to others still battling cancer. Long-term survivors meet newly diagnosed people and those newly gifted with remission news at those events. The American Brain Tumor Association has named its conferences "Sharing Hope."

Many communities participate in the growing movement, Relay for Life, sponsored by and benefiting the American Cancer Society. In more than 4,500 communities across the nation, teams of people camp out overnight—usually on a Friday—at local high school tracks, parks, or fairgrounds. Team members take turns walking around a track or path. Each team member raises money, seeking donations from individuals and businesses. Often there is friendly rivalry among teams striving to bring in the most money.

A Relay for Life evening usually begins with a Survivors' Walk, followed by a Caregivers' Walk. Participants usually wear special Relay for Life tee shirts. Relays raise funds for cancer research, but they are meant to be fun as well. Many teams adopt a slogan for their group and create costumes illustrating the theme. Sometimes, team members enjoy a potluck supper before setting out on their walking adventures. Our community relay holds a silent auction with items donated by local businesses. Community spirit and camaraderie prevail. Many friendships are begun and strengthened at these events.

Each team is to have a team representative walking the track at all times during this overnight event. The all-night representation is symbolic: cancer never sleeps. When the sun goes down, hundreds of luminaries line the track, lighting the way under the stars to remember those lost to cancer, those still battling cancer, and those who have fought and won. The luminaries lighting up the night symbolize the hope with which we all continue to fight—for ourselves and for others. Beginning at dusk and going well into the night, a list of names taken from the luminaries is read aloud. As twilight gives way to darkness, the crowd of spectators dwindles and quiet settles over the walkers. Nothing is heard but the continuous reading aloud of the names.

Another fundraising effort, Angel Adventure, supports brain tumor research and patient services. Sponsored by the National Brain Tumor Association, the 5K walk is designed for both teams and individuals. A half-day community event, Angel Adventure is relatively new, presently limited to communities in Arizona, California, and Colorado. You can find information about this fundraiser on the National Brain Tumor Foundation Web site.

One of the most surprising elements of survival is finding a new direction, using a latent or previously underutilized talent. David Bailey is an inspiring example of career turnaround. When diagnosed with a Grade IV GBM in 1996, he left a corporate position and, using his talents and musical background, he is now an inspiration and a joy to anyone who has experienced cancer and to all who love to listen to music.

The songs that Bailey plays and sings tell a story of conquering overwhelming odds. He writes his own music and lyrics, fashioned in the style of legendary folk singers, producing a combination uniquely Bailey. A David Bailey performance or CD carries a touch of poignancy and a dash of humor, overlaid with a strong dose of hope and love of life. He is seldom home, as his new calling keeps him on tour, away from his home in Virginia, much of the year. To his family, Bailey says, "This is what Daddy does."

David Bailey's present success was not achieved overnight. Like most brain cancer people, he has walked through the proverbial fire and—like iron turned to steel—come out stronger. As with many brain tumors, Bailey's tumor presented with excruciating headaches. After he "fell over one morning," emergency surgery removed a baseball-size tumor. His surgeon was not optimistic about chances for long-term survival, a fact unacceptable to Bailey. After searching the Internet and talking to people involved in various clinical trials, he contacted Dr. Henry Friedman at Duke University. At that time, David Bailey was thirty years old.

Trust built between patient and physician immediately, and Bailey says they found a way to face the facts, and then moved on to tackle the emotional, intellectual, and spiritual needs of the situation. At that time, Temodar was still a promising new drug in clinical trials. But, says Bailey, "It worked for me." After completing the trial and preparing for radiation, he was diagnosed with another low-grade tumor, which had to be surgically removed. Six weeks of radiation therapy followed the surgery. No new tumors would appear, a port was installed in the tumor bed, and a monoclonal antibody treatment was initiated.

All went well for almost six months, and then MRI showed the need for more chemotherapy. When a biopsy showed necrosis (dead tumor tissue) Bailey knew the battle had been won, but to be certain, doctors prescribed one more drug, followed by tamoxifen, a hormone therapy generally given to breast cancer patients that has shown promise in the treatment of brain tumors. Presently, David Bailey enjoys clear MRI scans, but small seizures continue to be a problem, along with some balance issues and limited peripheral vision. He says he tires quickly and is a bit slow when suddenly switching topics. When asked how he copes with the issue of fatigue, he is quick to answer, "Naps."

After a cancer journey that brought him to edge of death more than once, the fact that he celebrates life with his music illustrates what he says put his life back on track: faith in God, family, and friends and new windows and doors opening to a new future. David Bailey's Web site is listed in the appendix.

Bob Blum was enjoying a high-level career with the city of Houston, Texas, when, at the age of fifty-eight, he suffered a grand mal seizure. No other symptoms had presented, and Bob says that prior to the seizure he had enjoyed excellent health. MRI showed a tumor in the right temporal lobe. After some discussion, he was admitted to M. D. Anderson Cancer Center, where he underwent surgery, radiation, and a protocol that included intrathecal infusions (chemotherapy through an Ommaya reservoir). Unlike some whose brain cancer announced itself in a life changing fashion, Bob was able to continue working while being treated, except for the days he received chemotherapy as a hospital patient.

Prior to brain cancer, Bob was a practicing Jew. He says that during his first radiation treatment, Jesus found him. There was a great light, and then the face of Jesus appeared. Bobby Blum now calls himself a Messianic Jew, referring to Old Testament Bible prophecies declaring Yeshua of Nazareth (Jesus Christ) to be the Messiah. Messianic Jews remain true to their Jewish heritage and values while maintaining strong Christian beliefs. Bobby says that God wanted him to stay around for a purpose.

After recovery from primary CNS non-Hodgkin's lymphoma, Bobby attended training classes for lay chaplaincy work. Now he volunteers almost full time, traveling between several hospitals in the Houston area to visit with and counsel cancer patients and their families.

Bobby chuckles when he remembers meeting a man at Willowbrook Methodist Hospital who calls himself a Messianic Jew. "He came at it from the other side," says Bobby, explaining that the man had been a Christian who expanded to accept and practice "the Jewish ways as Jesus." Bobby poses the question: Where would the Old Testament be without the New Testament in the Bible and vice versa? Brain cancer, says Bobby, had made him "a fisher of men."

Like many brain cancer survivors, Bobby Blum says that his biggest frustration is difficulty with short-term memory. But, he says, brain cancer has changed him spiritually and emotionally. His pace has slowed, partly due to the fatigue that many survivors face and partly because he now recognizes the importance of God's gifts shown in everyday events. Now he likes to "listen to the sound of the sun going down."

Brain tumor survivors share their stories in many venues. Recently, University Hospital in Colorado began a tradition of holding cancer survivor dinners and celebrations for which people are encouraged to write their stories for display. The Brain Tumor Society encourages survivors and caregivers to send in their stories or coping hints for publication in the society's quarterly bulletin. Nothing is as sweet as those four words: You are in remission. It makes you want to shout it from the housetops. You have your life back, but there lingers the question: Why do I survive while others do not? It is a very human reaction and addresses a question for which there is no answer. What you do with your life after facing death may surprise you.

Chapter 11
Rebuilding the Body

During a cancer battle, the weeks and months of struggle take their toll on the body. I grew to think of this period in my husband's cancer journey as the mop-up operation. The body has suffered an assault, both from the cancer and from the treatments. The oncology team had saved his life, and he emerged with a triumphant spirit but with a weakened body and a great load of fatigue. My caregiver role expanded once again with the realization that I had more to learn.

Part of the body restoration project involves realistic thinking: accepting the need to pace oneself and learning the art of listening to one's own body. This is part of rebuilding life around a new normal. I brought up the issue of fatigue and side effects from chemotherapy with a medical professional one evening in a support group meeting. Doctors are so intent on saving lives that they frequently overlook the long-term effects of treatment. Fortunately, those involved in cancer treatments and rehabilitation issues are beginning to acknowledge and address the problems that surface in post-cancer life. More choices for follow-up care are becoming available and more easily accessible, and more information is becoming available.

For example, the National Cancer Institute, under the umbrella of the U.S. National Institutes of Health (NIH), conducts research through the Office of Cancer Survivorship, established in 1996. Part of its mission is to disseminate information to help guide cancer survivors through the first days or weeks following completion of treatment. The free booklet *Facing Forward: Life after Cancer* gives practical ways of dealing with common problems and offers guidelines for managing physical, social, and emotional health. To obtain a copy, you can call 1-800-4-CANCER or go to www.cancer.gov/cancertopics/life-after-treatment.

The Brain Tumor Society points out that fatigue after a brain tumor is not only treatment related but due to the "insult" caused by the tumors. It is normal to feel tired after treatments have ended. Fatigue may be due to reduced nutritional intake during chemotherapy. If food doesn't taste right or the idea of eating produces nausea, you may need to consult a dietician or nutritionist to help plan a better pattern of eating. Even if pre-cancer life allowed a person to thrive on little sleep each night, survivors need more sleep after brain cancer. It is important to avoid becoming impatient if energy does not seem to return quickly. The disease took a long time to appear and to be treated. As with any serious, debilitating disease, energy returns gradually. Moreover, the process of regaining energy doesn't usually progress in orderly fashion; what is possible to accomplish one day may be impossible another day. The trick is to look back over a chunk of time encompassing weeks or months. Improvements are gauged by looking at a broader picture. After coming so far in this battle, caregivers and their loved ones need not become discouraged.

Regaining physical strength often requires the assistance of a physical therapist, preferably one trained in working with cancer survivors. A physical therapist guides you through exercises to increase muscle strength and endurance. Physical therapy did much to improve my husband's quality of life. Because of the paralysis in his right arm before diagnosis, the shoulder muscles had tightened and locked into place, making it impossible to raise his arm above a certain level. Surgery was not an option in our view. The rehabilitation center near our home had proved its worth in our life the year before when I was recovering from the effects of Guillain Barre. So, without hesitation, we put George under Gil's care.

She concentrated her efforts on the right shoulder, with exercise and massage. Within a few weeks, full range of motion returned to the arm. Next, she worked on his legs. Gaining leg strength and eliminating painful neuropathy brought on by the chemotherapy has been a long project, but we press on. Water therapy—exercising in the heated pool at the rehabilitation center—has been helpful. Warm water helps relax tight muscles, and moving about in water creates just the right amount of resistance without straining muscles.

A physical therapist goes through the exercises with you and then makes sure you will know how to conduct them on your own. The "homework" is diagramed on a sheet of paper. For water therapy, George received a set of laminated, waterproof cards. After formal therapy is completed (or the insurance company decides you don't need any more therapy), people can continue the exercises on their own. Many community pools are heated, and some rehabilitation centers open their pools to the public at specified hours.

Cancer rehabilitation centers offer comprehensive programs of various therapies designed especially for people recovering from the effects of cancer. An example of this growing movement is Navitas, the nation's first independent network of outpatient cancer rehabilitation clinics. Whether one chooses an independent clinic or one affiliated with a hospital or cancer center, therapists and other staff are trained to deal with the unique needs of cancer survivors. Most survivors want to continue strengthen activities after formal therapy is completed. Yoga and tai chi classes, available at community recreation centers or private fitness centers, also provide a good way to relax, regain movement, and meet others with the same goal.

For ongoing physical problems in post-cancer life, acupuncture might be a viable option. My husband's biggest problem after treatments ended was neuropathy (degeneration of the peripheral nerves). His legs and feet felt and performed like lead blocks. Part of the problem was a residual of the chemotherapy drugs and part was damage incurred from the tumors pressing on part of the brain. During the time that the four large tumors were growing inside his brain, George experienced discomfort in his feet, gradually worsening to the point where walking barefoot across carpeting caused acute pain. In addition, before diagnosis and continuing after treatment ended, there was weakness and loss of balance, along with the feeling of walking on rocks. Pain breeds pain; that is, pain breaks down our defenses to the point where muscles tighten and the entire body braces itself against remembered pain. This constant defense mode results in lessened activity, which then allows muscles to atrophy. Such was the case with George. Before the problem was brought under control, he had lost even more muscle tone.

Some of the remediation from foot pain resulted from George's inventiveness as well as therapy. Part of rehabilitation involved nerve stimulation, with the therapist using several different modalities. At home, George grew into the habit of massaging his feet twice a day, concentrating especially on the soles of his feet, where the feeling had been most affected.

Years later, the damage from neuropathy is not completely gone, but we have achieved distinct improvement. It has been a long, hard process, but the shuffling gait has disappeared. George's legs do not allow him to run or even walk fast, but they have come back to a more normal function. We owe much of the improvement to acupuncture, periodic visits to a clinic that offers relief for various problems, using traditional Chinese medicine.

Toward the end of George's protocol, his feet grew ice cold, taking on a bluish-white tinge. Already comfortable with our local practitioner, knowing that acupuncture is not an invasive procedure, and knowing what to expect during an appointment, we scheduled a visit at the clinic. One treatment brought startling results. Proper circulation brought adequate blood flow through the legs and to the feet, resulting in healthy color and warmer skin. According to traditional Chinese medicine, the energy channels (*qi*, pronounced "chee") were blocked.

Now, years later, my husband visits an acupuncturist for what I call a "tune-up." As our insurance company does not cover such treatments, we have to address the issue of cost. We are fortunate to live near an acupuncture college that offers reduced rates with third-year students working under supervision of credentialed Chinese doctors.

Acupuncture is also becoming more readily available outside the realm of Chinese medicine as physicians trained in Western medicine join the trend toward integrated medicine. Centers for Integrative Medicine can be found in many communities. Complementary and Alternative Medicine (CAM) includes treatment with herbs, massage, acupuncture, and diet counseling. The National Cancer Institute Web site offers information on some CAM therapies of interest to cancer survivors. Some physicians trained in conventional medical practices have also become certified to practice acupuncture. If you choose that approach, be sure to ask how many hours of instruction and practice the doctor has completed. The American Academy of Medical Acupuncture requires a minimum of 200 hours graduate training in Medical Acupuncture.

Acupuncture is not always a permanent cure, but used periodically it can provide relief from pain and add needed energy. Many insurance companies do not pay for acupuncture treatments performed by anyone other than a doctor trained primarily in conventional medicine. This restriction ignores the fact that a licensed practitioner of traditional Chinese medicine has been required to pass rigorous exams after three thousand hours of class work and clinical experience, including use of herbal medicines, massage, acupressure, and acupuncture—all done under close supervision of instructors licensed and experienced in the art of traditional Chinese medicine.

Typically, the first time you see a practitioner, an acupuncture appointment will take ninety minutes or more, including the time during which the practitioner inquires about your eating and sleeping habits, takes your pulse on each wrist, and examines your tongue. The tongue is a key indicator as to the state of your health and the treatment you will require. Sometimes part of the procedure will include moxibustion, a type of weed grown in China, dried and used as a heat application. The smoke that is generated has a sharp, acrid odor, described by some as similar to the odor of marijuana.

Acupuncture is, of course, associated with the use of needles, and some people can't visualize themselves lying on a table with a couple of dozen or more needles in their body. However, acupuncture needles used in the United States are quite slender. A skilled acupuncturist can insert needles so quickly and painlessly that the patient need only lie still and relax. Massage and acupressure may be included in an appointment as well. Many practitioners play soft music during treatments.

In addition to acupuncture, George's battle with neuropathy has included the use of vitamin supplements. Vitamin B_{12} and amino acids play a large part of our nutrition planning. On his doctor's recommendation, George tried vitamin D to reduce the nighttime shooting pains and cramps in legs and feet. The doctor also warned us that the statin drug George was taking to reduce cholesterol might be a contributing factor to his sleep-disturbing leg cramps.

Living with neuropathy can be challenging, but there are many things that people can do in everyday care. For example, regularly massaging the bottoms of nerve-damaged feet will alleviate pain and boost circulation. Wearing pads inside shoes helps to cushion the bottoms of tender feet. Gel pads are available and reasonably priced at discount stores and pharmacies. George wears good quality athletic shoes for all occasions except for events that call for a more formal look. Regular dress shoes are too stiff for his feet and cause discomfort, making them inappropriate for long periods.

Peripheral neuropathy can also bring loss of balance. George's sense of balance was compromised early in the cancer journey because of the location of the brain tumors, and that deficit will be with him always. During treatment and for several months afterward, he used a cane for help with balance while walking. If the doctor cautions against climbing ladders, take the advice seriously. As time passes and the period of diagnosis and treatment fades into memory, a survivor may be tempted to take chances that put the body in jeopardy. Try to remember that you and your loved one have been through too much to risk harming the body any further.

Anyone with peripheral neuropathy has experienced the phenomena of exercising or doing some kind of physical work, then feeling pain and fatigue the next day or even several days later. A person with damaged nerves needs to be as careful with energy as if it were money in the bank: it is unwise to overdraw an energy account. This precaution is easier to talk about than it is to practice, but it is part of life in remission that needs to be built into the new lifestyle. My husband and I once attempted to tour all of Orlando, Florida's immense Epcot Center on foot—a foolhardy endeavor even for the able-bodied. Fortunately, the park, like many public attractions, offers wheelchairs for rent. Wheelchairs, electric scooters, and other devices are becoming more commonplace as people with physical limitations enjoy more of what the world has to offer outside the boundaries of home.

Survivors who desire to remain active while living with pain, weakness, and fatigue may want to obtain a handicap placard for the car. In most states, the placard goes along with the driver or passenger, so if you are on a trip and will be renting a car, you can take your handicap placard along. In our state, the placard needs to be renewed every three years, an easy process. Getting an initial handicap permit entails picking up a form at the driver license office, filling it out, and having the doctor sign it. Our handicap placard has saved a lot of pain and inconvenience.

Another part of our mop-up operation has addressed the issue of eyesight. The damage that occurred when tumors were pressing on George's optic nerve has created the need for special glasses with built-in prisms to correct the double vision that originally signaled the presence of brain tumors. Our ophthalmologist has to prescribe new glasses every year, and field of vision is monitored on a regular basis. It's another segment of body management after cancer and necessary for maintaining quality of life.

Living within the range of a "new normal" might be frustrating at times. You and your loved one are trying to keep what level of health is left, nurturing the hope that there is improvement with time. Everyone recovers at a different pace and within a different timeframe, so avoid comparing progress with other survivors.

Both George and I live with a degree of physical limitation that makes walking or hiking long distances difficult if not impossible. One day, while visiting with friends, the subject of exercise came up. "Last week we rode our bicycles fifty miles up to the mountains and back," one man boasted. I churned inside, longing to say that I would have been happy to ride one mile, or even to balance myself on a bicycle. A glance at George told me that he had the same thought. People don't always think before they talk. We can either point out the error of their comments or remain silent, depending on the circumstances and our preferences.

Friends and acquaintances don't mean to hurt our feelings; most people have not traveled the path we have journeyed and do not realize what we have had to overcome. Unless a person is in a wheelchair, wearing leg braces, or exhibiting some other visible sign of disability, the average observer does not realize the limitations. People with invisible handicaps endure loss of credibility every day.

George, like many cancer survivors, tells others of the miracle of his healing every chance he has. "But you look so good now," is the most common reaction. It must be the sparkle in his eyes, and his love of life after having come so close to losing it.

Chapter 12
Regaining the Use of a
Damaged Brain

An article from the December 2001 issue of *OconoLog,* published on the M. D. Anderson Web site, states that "cognitive impairments may result from the cancer itself or from neurotoxic side effects of cancer treatments...." Years ago, little thought was given to what sort of life a brain cancer survivor would experience after being pronounced in remission. Without the advanced techniques and sophisticated equipment that have become available in the last few years, few patients survived brain cancer. Now, people diagnosed with brain cancer are surviving and living productive, albeit changed, lives.

Brain cancer does more than leave an impact on the body; tumors in the brain may leave brain damage and the treatments leave their mark as well. During the period of treatment, doctors concentrate on saving lives, but give scant attention to possible cognitive deficits after remission. The question of cognitive rehabilitation has been largely ignored until recently, but increased survival rates have impelled researchers to evaluate the quality-of-life issues that brain tumor survivors and their families face. Ongoing neuropsychological studies are being conducted to provide information about treatment toxicity and how it affects quality of life in brain cancer survivors. The three large non-profit brain tumor groups are doing much to address the issue of cognitive rehabilitation, offering information regarding neuropsychological testing and explaining the rehabilitation process.

The National Brain Tumor Foundation has published a fact sheet, written by Sandra M. Portman, Ph.D., that lists six common difficulties brain tumor survivors experience involving mind, emotion, and personality. Brain tumor patients, she says, show different patterns and progressions than other patients affected by neurological conditions, such as stroke or head trauma. Damage done by brain tumors is different from other types of brain injury, and rehabilitation programs must consider that difference when planning treatment. In addition to damage created by edema when the tumors are growing and pressing on parts of the brain, the brain sustains injury during surgery, radiation, immunotherapy, and chemotherapy. Often, the changes evolve so gradually that caregivers and health providers barely notice.

Portman advises brain tumor survivors to contact their physicians for help in choosing a neuropsychologist, a professional who specializes in cognitive evaluation and rehabilitation. If possible, says Portman, try to find a neuropsychologist who has experience in working specifically with brain tumor survivors. Other avenues to explore would include vocational rehabilitation, job coaches in the work setting, and individual psychotherapy.

The American Brain Tumor Association offers information through the article "Cognitive Retraining," part of the "Becoming Well Again Through …" quality-of-life series. Cognitive rehabilitation concentrates both on learning a cognitive skill such as planning or problem solving and on developing strategies to compensate for impaired ability. The article suggests activities such as workbooks, puzzles, board games, and problem solving on various levels. Strategies to improve memory, develop organization skills, and avoid confusion are included as well. The authors urge patience. The brain needs time to heal, and it needs time and practice to develop new ways to do things you once accomplished with little effort.

Understandably, brain tumor survivors may become frustrated with the process of healing a damaged brain. The Brain Tumor Society offers the COPE (Connection of Personal Experiences) program. As with other cancer hot lines, volunteers offer support through sharing of mutual experiences via e-mail and telephone conversations. Just as in support group settings, the idea is to reduce the feeling of isolation. As the volunteers are also cancer survivors, the benefits of communication are mutual. The director of COPE is Sarah Gupta, LICSW. You can reach her at 800-770-8287, ext 25, or support@tbs.org.

As part of follow-up care, your physician may recommend neuropsychological testing—a detailed series of tests measuring cognitive deficits in the areas of orientation to time and place, the ability to repeat and then remember new information, the ability for sustained attention, the ability to use language, and the ability to copy a simple drawing. Neuropsychologists are trained to administer IQ tests and tests to identify brain injuries and altered cognitive functions. A neuropsychologist will use the results of your tests and plan a program that might include speech therapy and occupational therapy as well as cognitive treatment and assistance in overcoming depression. Dr. Malcom P. Rogers, a psychiatrist at Brigham and Women's Hospital in Boston, Massachusetts, and a member of the advisory board of the Brain Tumor Society, states that information about cognitive function helps loved ones to understand the confusion and frustration of brain tumor survivors struggling with neurological damage.

Speech and language pathologists are important components of recovery from a brain tumor. These specialists address the issue of speech difficulties and memory loss. Difficulty with memory varies with individuals, but in general, there are three different stages of memory: learning stage, storage stage, and recall stage. All three of these stages are affected by brain tumors. Stress and anxiety can hamper rehabilitation; brain tumor survivors can become depressed and frustrated over elusive memories and compromised cognitive abilities, so it's important that everyone involved in the healing process remain calm and confident.

Speech-language pathologist Jill Newcombe at the University Hospital in Colorado recommends focusing on one task at a time and working in a quiet environment to avoid becoming distracted and confused. Making lists and writing things down is helpful. A sense of humor is a great leveler. It's hard to worry while laughing. My husband and I developed our own mini-skit. When he would make a mistake or experience difficulty remembering something, he would say, "What do you expect? I had four brain tumors." To which I would retort, "I can't think good either. I'm married to someone with a brain tumor." Such repartee may not strike a humorous note with people outside the brain tumor community, but it got us through many tense moments. To help keep a healthy perspective on our difficulties, it's important to remember that even people with no cognitive problems experience occasional memory lapses.

Restoring memory and rebuilding cognitive abilities take time and patience, with or without the help of professionals. When my husband was pronounced in remission, we did not immediately take time to research all the elements of available support, remaining content to focus on living one day at a time, with a sense of release, like two small children who had been told they could have their birthday party after all. When the radiology report showed that the four viable tumors had been reduced to dead (necrotic) tissue, our relief was so great that all we cared about was celebrating, doing all the things we'd put on hold during the nightmare weeks of battling cancer. We did not wish to look back.

Eventually, euphoria gave way to reality and George began the daunting task of recreating his memory bank and rebuilding his ability to think. For years, his engineering background and inherent logic skills had enabled him to solve complex problems. Now he would embark on solving the largest problem of his life. My caregiver job was about to change. Instead of performing clearly defined tasks, such as taking notes at medical appointments and dispensing medication, I would need to apply different skills. I would be the backup thinker, the one who would gently remind him of details, possible consequences of certain actions or lack of actions. In short, I would be the proverbial woman behind the man. The prospect was daunting.

In this rehabilitation stage of the brain tumor journey, caregivers need to know when to encourage, when to push, and when to cease pushing their loved ones. Encouragement is needed for each small step forward. Patience is needed when there is a lull while preparing for the next attempt. Fear of failure is real, and the two of you need to set realistic goals, using small steps. Also, be aware that what might be achieved one day may be impossible to accomplish the next day. Recovery can be a recursive event—two steps forward and one step backward. That's OK; it takes time and much repetition to build new neuro pathways.

George referred to his lost memories when he would say that his "bridges were washed out." Indeed they were. Many of our conversations would begin with my saying, "Do you remember ...?" His curt retort: "No, I *don't* remember." Gradually, the negative would replace the positive and we could enter conversations about past events, trading pieces of information to create a patchwork quilt of our past. We were fortunate to have years of memories from our life together to draw upon.

Looking back on his state of mind during and immediately after treatment, George confides some startling facts about his feelings at that time. "With no memory, all fears are destroyed, and it's easy to have a cheerful expression on your face constantly. As long as you are fed and no longer need diapers or frequent changes of underwear, you are content and happy. But you are also living in a vacuum." Fortunately, I did not realize what a dark and empty place his mind had become until much later in our cancer journey. He has had to work hard to come back from the place he describes.

George now draws an analogy, comparing his lost memory to a very large city with a river running straight through the middle. For as long as the city existed, people could cross the river on any of more than a dozen bridges. Then, one day a tidal wave washed out all but one of the bridges. Huge traffic jams resulted as travelers from all over the city were forced to drive long distances to cross the one useable bridge; commerce between the two sides of the city slowed down, creating short tempers, frustration, and fatigue from the extra effort of driving long distances on crowded highways.

The issue of fatigue is foremost among brain tumor survivors. Short and long-term survivors in our support group admit to fatigue of one degree or another. Some days may be filled with more energy than others, but all those recovering from a brain tumor will need more sleep. The days are gone when my husband could get by with five or six hours of sleep each night for long periods. Eight to ten hours is now the ideal.

One evening our support group spent the whole meeting discussing the issue of fatigue. Once past the debilitating effects of chemotherapy and radiation and of the disease itself, why does fatigue linger like an unwanted guest at a party that concluded hours before? The feeling of exhaustion present in brain tumor survivors is unlike the tired feeling earned by hard physical exercise or even by lack of sleep. Expending mental energy means tapping into the power force of the mind. Searching for words, phrases, events, and ideas in the jumble left by brain tumors takes energy. I have watched survivors struggle to express themselves; words come slowly as they search through jumbled files that have not yet been resorted and organized. Participating in conversation or being in a classroom, or in some other group activity where one must pay close attention, burns precious energy. One caregiver revealed that during the period when he was receiving heavy doses of chemotherapy, her husband would visit his office and engage in stimulating conversation with his colleagues without missing a beat. Upon returning home, he would lie down, exhausted from expending mental energy. The stimulation of being in a large group of people or even participating in a one-on-one discussion can drain energy from a brain tumor survivor.

On the other hand, it is not a good idea to retreat from the rest of the world, avoiding group and learning situations altogether. The key is moderation and knowing one's own limits. Recovery of the mind takes tenacity and time. I have noticed George's vocabulary increase over time as his store of words gradually returns. It has taken many years to come to this state of recovery. Brain cancer attacks swiftly, brutally. The disease can be conquered, but the damage it leaves behind takes work and time to repair.

George looks back upon those days of when all that had happened in his life was a blank slate. He remembers wondering if he would ever function as a human being again. Reading was impossible. He could not recall the slightest detail of what he had read, heard, or learned just twenty-four hours before. A sentence is a complex construct, full of detail too complicated to decode for one who was, as he says, "functioning like an idiot." Unless he could see a picture of something, he could not process it. He could not remember longer than twenty-four hours the names and faces of people in our brain tumor support group; his only other contact with the world was our home and our church.

Gradually, George could retain information by focusing on one or two names and faces at a time, but no more. The brain would not tolerate overload. He could understand concepts, but details of any kind were out of reach for him. Many how-to books had accumulated in our household over the years he took care of all the maintenance on our cars, repaired large and small appliances as needed, planned and completed simple and complicated renovation projects, and created beautifully handcrafted items in wood. The books had been a source of inspiration and instruction, but now they were nothing to him, even if he could remember where they were. His reading skills had vanished, but he burned with a desire to relearn everything he could as quickly as possible.

One day, he recalled something told to him as a student at Brooklyn Technical High School: read a technical book three times in order to fully understand what it is saying. He then began to apply that concept in another, more visual fashion. We have always enjoyed the educational programs on public television, and before brain cancer George had taped many of the broadcasts. During this intense cognitive rehabilitation phase, he viewed those programs repeatedly until the visions were implanted in his memory.

He then expanded the repetition concept, watching a brief segment—sometimes as short as one sentence—of each video three times. In this way, he built up a store of new memories that then enabled new neuro pathways to expand. The "washed out bridges" were becoming new roads as the brain began its restoration. The process continues; for every new memory built, two more are released. Sometimes a whole flood of memories returns.

The miracle of cognitive recovery, however, is not without its difficulties. Short-term memory continues to be a problem, and I struggle to control my impatience when my husband cannot share a brief memory of some trivial incident that may have taken place the previous week or even the day before. On the other hand, visions of events from as long ago as fifty years suddenly appear in his mind.

While faulty memory is annoying and sometimes time consuming as we hunt, sometimes for hours, for misplaced objects, the ability to reason and predict consequences has been far more difficult to master. George says that his ability to think ahead and figure out logical steps in simple procedures was "about on the level of a three-year-old child." That deficit remained for months after completion of treatment, and traces of it linger to a small extent. Caregivers in these circumstances walk a fine line between nagging and reminding, but it was most encouraging to hear one of our grandsons admonish his grandpa that he is "lucky to have her." It is hard to remain humble under such praise.

A turning point in the battle to master thinking skills occurred one year after chemotherapy ended. During the long weeks of chemotherapy infusions, repeated blood draws, and trips to the hospital, George had dreamed of a fishpond in our back yard. I also imagined the soothing sounds of a waterfall and the cooling effect of a water feature just outside the kitchen door. The project turned out to be a combination of physical therapy and cognitive rehabilitation.

A local building supply store was closing out its season's supply of preformed plastic fishponds. The only sizes offered were extra big and extra small. The big ponds were beyond the scope of both George and me, and they would have been inappropriate for our tiny backyard. We bought a small pond shell—the fifty-gallon size. I had never been skilled in the art of conceptualizing and bringing to completion home improvement projects, so George was largely on his own, free to make mistakes and muddle through, learning as he progressed.

With no concept of size and with vague memories of the 750-gallon concrete shell pond he had built for our much larger yard thirty years before, George set about installing the 50-gallon plastic shell pond. He had listened carefully to the salesman's instructions and retained the first sentence: First, you dig a hole. After some maneuvering, George got the plastic shell to fit in the hole. Then, he remembered the salesman's admonition to put sand in the bottom of the hole. More maneuvering, then success—the shell fit into the hole. However, the edge of the plastic shell stood a couple of inches from the ground, requiring some adjustment in the level of the sand and the depth of the hole.

All this time, I had observed with increasing horror as once again I realized it was up to me to think ahead on situations involving projects and problem solving. No longer the stronger and more capable one, George needed my help with thinking. Brushing aside my anxieties, I regarded the plastic shell sitting in the hole and remembered the pond and waterfall we had enjoyed for so many years long ago. "What about electricity for the pump?" Noticing a questioning look, I persisted. "You know. Rocks for decoration and for the waterfall you wanted."

"Electricity? Rocks? Oh, I guess I'm not done."

There followed months of hard physical work on George's part. Lifting and carrying large rocks in the process of choosing, purchasing, and unloading them at home helped to rebuild muscles long unused. The mental challenges were enormous as George arranged and rearranged the rocks around the pond to create the effect we both wanted.

George says that words like "helpless" and "idiot" went through his head as he worked to stay focused on one small step at a time—building, tearing apart, and redoing over and over to complete a project that would have taken a weekend before the brain tumors appeared in our life. A couple of months later, we planted some flowers in the garden around the pond, and together we attended a class at a local nursery on pond maintenance.

With each small accomplishment, George's comfort level rose, and he gained confidence to approach new challenges. He remembered watching our grandchildren learning to walk and to master tasks. If they could learn, he could learn also. Most of his effort toward learning was modeled on the way babies learn. He knew he was dependent on others' reasoning ability, and he was determined to learn and do his best no matter how long it took. I doubt if I would have had the patience and persistence to complete a task as formidable as that pond must have appeared to George.

Since overcoming that first big challenge, other smaller but no less formidable tasks remained. Many still linger. For months the little garage workshop where George ran a small business—building custom-designed computers—stood unused and cluttered with the remnants of his last work days before brain cancer brought productivity to a halt. A quick glance at computer parts and software mingled with sales brochures, e-mail messages, old receipts, and technical periodicals gave the impression of a place where a battle had been fought and lost.

"Someday," George would say, "I will get organized." He saw himself as a cripple and harbored serious doubts of getting back to an acceptable level of functioning. He prayed for the strength to persevere, to meet the challenge. I watched and waited for my husband to come back from his dark place of confusion with only my childlike faith in God for support.

When he set about to recall his past life and the things he had learned in all his years, he knew enough to realize the task was enormous. Those were gloomy days. One day, several months after we heard the glorious news of remission, the celebratory mood had leveled off and I had gone back to work, leaving George alone in the house for large portions of the day. Wishing to communicate his feelings of love for family and devotion to God, he sat at the computer and prayed for words to express his feelings.

When I returned home at the end of the day, a triumphant husband showed me what he had done. George had completed a two-page story describing the miracle of his cancer journey and all that had been important in his life. The skill of manipulating words to create sentences and using sentences to communicate ideas had returned. Other cancer survivors and those just beginning their battle have referred to the story as inspiring. Writing it was the first big step in recovery.

Even before brain cancer, George learned in a visual manner; using that strength has been the key to building new memories. After brain cancer, this method has been the key to a self-education project that has opened the door to subjects he previously ignored for lack of time. He calls these expanding interests one of the "blessings of cancer." No longer limited to reading technical publications or instructions for do-it-yourself projects, George has branched out into studying the non-technical subjects not emphasized while earning his electrical engineering degree. As his strongest mode of learning is through visual aids, he delves into history and travel videos with the same tenacity that powered his rehabilitation.

George can repair computers again. He has even built a couple of machines for our grandchildren. The work goes slowly. He pushes himself and works with painstaking attention to details, lest they elude him. He has to proceed through each phase of a job, using trial and error, reeducating himself on the latest technology and relying on technical support hotlines for assistance in working through each step of the job. As with the pond project, he forges ahead through mistakes and repetition, but each victory brings courage and confidence.

We have grown accustomed to hearing acquaintances remark on how well George appears after they hear about his brush with death and subsequent recovery. Many people are curious about the transformation from severe cognitive loss to the level of improvement that allows our quality of life. They ask how George managed to recover from such a deteriorated state.

Our answer is that we asked for and received the help of God. George prayed for to regain the use of language and logic. I prayed for the strength to live two lives—his and mine—for the period during which George was finding his way back. Much of the time, I didn't feel up to the job. I didn't allow myself to ponder the future, during treatment and during the intense rehabilitation phase. But cancer has been a blessing for me also, in that I have gained strength I never realized I had.

Rebuilding the "bridges" continues. As each memory returns, something else is triggered and a new chain of thought is begun. More and larger chunks of thought appear, and recall becomes easier every day. George says that remembering past accomplishments has helped a lot: a basic "grid" has emerged that helps him to function efficiently but slowly, concentrating on one problem at a time. Cognitive irregularities remain, increasing and decreasing on a daily or even hourly basis, depending on the demands of the moment and current level of energy. Life after brain cancer is not the same, and we are traveling a far different path than anyone ever plans for, but life is good.

Chapter 13
Sharing Hope

Throughout our cancer journey, we have learned quite a bit about listening to God, a habit that had previously required more patience than I was prepared to apply. When George prayed, asking God to grant him four extra weeks on Earth (added to the twelve weeks hoped for by the medical team), he expected God to hear him, and he did. I, on the other hand, harbored no such expectations; my mind at that time contained no greater vision than a long, black tunnel that I must travel each day without thought or feeling.

By going through each day, each moment, without thought of the future, I survived the time of my husband's cancer treatments. Before we had obtained definite diagnosis, a false sense of hope alternating with a defensive posture of denial instilled in me the erroneous thought that any day we would discover that all of George's problems were due to something tests had overlooked, something that could be easily fixed. A simple operation, a dose of medication, and all would be well again; such is the thinking of a desperate woman who does not know how to hope. My method of hoping could be called magical thinking, a form of twisted logic convincing me that because I wanted a simple and quick resolution to our dilemma a solution would appear and all would be well.

Diagnosis of brain tumor knocked the breath out of me; as a boxer receiving one punch too many staggers to his corner, resting for another round, I retreated inside myself to gather strength. The days ahead would require endurance, something I'd been short on since recovering from debilitating illness myself. GuillainBarre, I told myself, is nothing. I lived through it. Most people stricken with that disease survive, but brain cancer takes away lives. I resolved to hold on to my husband's life through sheer will power if nothing else. He could not die. He would not die. However, the protocol was well underway before I would admit to God and to myself the terror I was keeping at bay by staying busy with mindless tasks.

So I concentrated on the immediate jobs, tangible things that could be accomplished with physical effort. The previous year I had experienced being cared for, and now it was my turn to care. Keeping my husband alive would become my single most important project. My illness of a short time before would give me the ability to recognize the needs and feelings of a patient; with the roles reversed, I would have empathy. I would know what to do. That bravado lasted a very short time; George's ordeal would be nothing like mine of the previous year. I had to reinvent the script.

Only until a plan for treatment began to form did I gain a small measure of control over the small daily events. Even then, each day—each hour—presented challenges. Any thought or plan beyond the immediate present continued in my mind as an enormous void. By keeping busy with chores that required little or no planning or thought, I pushed myself through the days with one goal: getting our lives back to normal. If anyone had informed me that there would never be a normal, as we had always known it, I would have turned away and refused to listen. I needed time to accept what was going on, and taking baby steps or standing in place was the way I had of venturing into the future.

After the long period of George's gradual lapse into helplessness, circumstances that put him into the hands of skilled neurosurgeon and a competent pathologist were truly the first of God's many gifts during that summer of our brain cancer. The size and location of the four tumors dictated that there was no time to search for the best doctor, the right treatment center. Fortunately, by God's grace, we happened to be where we were supposed to be for the care George needed to have.

In *Making Miracles Happen,* Greg Smith talks about patients who show a "strange aversion to pursuing the best medical care, no matter how grave the consequences." Smith's conclusion that for some patients, traveling to search out more and better choices for treatment adds one more unknown factor to an already precarious situation. When we are seriously ill, he says, the tendency is to stay within familiar surroundings—to stay home where family and friends are near. That definition applied to George and me. Any idea of leaving home and traveling further than the big university hospital a few miles away seemed no more feasible than a trip to the moon. To me, the hospital where diagnosis occurred was the place where treatment should begin, and the sooner the better.

Reading that passage in Greg Smith's book has caused me to reflect on the crisis we faced in 1998. I thought about the months of symptoms, appearing one by one, gradually chipping away at George's quality of life until he was living at little more than the level of a small child—a suffering small child in an old man's body. All the while, I watched, helpless, as his movements grew slower and more obviously painful. With every visit to each different doctor—his primary care physician, the thyroid specialist, the doctor presiding over a colonoscopy that showed no reason for his digestive problems, the first ophthalmologist who could find no reason for the double vision—discouragement, frustration, and panic grew. *Please, God, let us know what is taking over his body. Let us know what to do and how to fight.* Brain cancer never entered the realm of possibility. I would settle for something that could be cut away, treated with a bit of medicine, and abolished from our lives. Then all would be well again. I had no idea that the hope I nurtured was misplaced, but lessons in hope would be forthcoming.

Always, suffering, sharing, and surviving boils down to a quest for hope, the element with which humanity obtains its existence. Hope means different things to various people. The dictionary puts the definition of hope succinctly: desire accompanied by expectation. The desire is there, but the expectation must also be clear. As the women who came to our home for the healing service that June day in 1998 asked George what he wanted to pray for, so God asks us to talk to him about our needs and expectations. That is when the healing service crystallized hope—for George and for me—into something solid, offering an attainable goal. I remembered something I'd heard long ago: With God all things are possible.

When George wrote his story during the cognitive rehabilitation portion of his transition into our new normal, he included two incidents from his boyhood that have influenced his faith in the power of prayer. One day, in a desperate situation, he called upon God for help. Like many families during the Depression, money was tight, but his mother had managed to purchase a Boy Scout hat, crucial for joining the local troop. While hiking in the woods, he lost the hat.

After hours of searching, he called upon God, who probably wondered why he had not been summoned before the search. When George finished praying, he opened his eyes and discovered the object he had hunted for with desperation and panic all day. One more miracle occurred months later when he lost a purse with the entire week of family grocery money. Once more, George offered up a plea for help and once more, he experienced God's protection when the purse was found shortly thereafter. Those two incidents formed a solid foundation of faith and hope that would enable him to withstand the brutal effects of treatment and the despair that sometimes overtakes the desperately ill.

In the "Miracle of Prayer," George cautions readers to be specific in their prayer requests but to "be prepared that some of the answers may not be what you want to hear." The story he wrote in 1998 goes on to say, "God expects us to see past the bad times that life (and perhaps Satan) can throw at us, to ask for God's help as He sees fit, and to never lose faith in God or to blame Him because He chose not to control us like robots."

Several weeks after suddenly regaining the use of language, George wrote another page, "Cancer: Improving Your Odds for Survival." The story of Job, the man in the Old Testament who lost everything, illustrates that faith in God during bad times allows us to put our lives in perspective. As with Job, George says, God gave me back twice what we had asked for. Cancer was a blessing, he says. "It helped me put my life in perspective, with time left to share my thoughts with family and friends." Now we share those written pages with anyone who asks how he was healed from brain cancer when all evidence showed it would not be possible.

Researchers are working on solving the puzzle of why some people live through brain cancer and its abusive treatments while others do not survive, but at this time there is no clear answer. We have known people who have prayed and been prayed for, asking God to take away the cancer and let them live awhile longer. We have seen their discouragement and the grief of their loved ones when the cancer returns or refuses to disappear. Worse, we have seen cancer patients angry with God for his seeming refusal to answer prayers for good health. My heart goes out to anyone who feels that prayer has been a wasted effort. No one can answer for God's mysterious ways. Our prayers for brain cancer, or any cancer, must first place the decision on the shoulders of our Creator, asking only for peace and for his will to be done. Anger must be saved to fight the cancer cells that destroy the body.

The September 2004 edition of *Christianity Today* features an article by Mark M. Yarbrough of Dallas Theological Seminary, addressing the issue of unanswered prayer. God, says Yarbrough, does not always respond to our desires in our timeframe. Because our requests do not always coincide with God's response, we interpret his silence as refusal to answer our prayers. Although we may look for affirmation of our faith in "signs and wonders," God does his finest work in circumstances and events that we may not comprehend. Yarbrough points out that the God of our joys is also the God of our sorrows, walking with us in the valley of shadows.

In another perspective, Rabbi Harold Kushner's 1981 bestseller attempts to explain why God appears to abandon good people. *When Bad Things Happen to Good People* points out, "Laws of nature do not make exceptions for nice people." And, says Kushner, things that happen because of our free will or as a result of natural phenomena are not because of God. God, he says, "does not reach down to interrupt the workings of laws of nature to protect the righteous from harm." However, we all have the gift of prayer, which can help us sustain the gift of hope.

In addition to expecting a desire to be fulfilled, hope involves a sense of control. If we feel in control of a situation, the sense of helplessness cannot prevail. Helplessness leads to despair, then loss of hope, and ultimately loss of life. Studies have been done with rats to prove this theory. Greg Smith writes of an experiment done by Madelon Baronoski, now a professor of psychology at Yale University. One group of rats was given electric shocks at random, uncontrollable intervals. Another group of rats was given electric shocks, but the rats were taught a way to control the shocks. All the rats were injected with cancer cells. Those who were subjected to shocks they could not control suffered a death rate of 75 to 80 percent. The second group, with the power to control the shocks, showed only a 25 percent death rate.

For most people, a diagnosis of brain cancer makes the world spin out of control. However, loss of control results in one becoming a victim. Cancer survivors and their loved ones are not victims but warriors. I was not able to pull together my resolve to help my husband fight until the pathology report confirmed the diagnosis and the treatment team outlined the protocol. Before that time, I was like a lost soul, adrift on a raft with no way to steer, at the mercy of wherever riptides and rapids would take me.

I remember struggling with my feelings when Dr. Schultz entered the hospital room and outlined the situation, explaining the options and consequences of each potential course of action. My panic deepened as it became evident that radiation therapy would do George more harm than good. Dr. Schultz explained each detail and described every possibility in a voice so gentle and compassionate that I knew he was sharing our grief. I fastened on the one choice that offered a small shred of hope—the aggressive treatment plan of high-dose chemotherapy. Dr. Schultz didn't pressure us to decide at that moment. He gave us time to absorb the information and he offered prayer support for whatever choice we would make.

Finally, the choice should always be up to the patient, once he or she knows all the options and has shared the decision with loved ones. George chose chemotherapy, with a dose so strong that he might not live through the treatments. He wanted the doctors to do whatever necessary to save his body, but he did not want to live without his mind. He'd had enough of confusion and frustration from inability to communicate clearly. The choice was a dangerous route in the short term, but it offered more hope for recovery without serious, permanent neurological deficits in the long term. I knew we had a plan—a project to work on. We both knew that the outcome was in God's hands, and that he would be with us every step of the way. George says that he felt he was in a win-win situation. Either he would die and go to heaven or he would live to enjoy his family and life itself for a while longer. In that mindset, we were in control. Cancer would not win, no matter what the outcome.

Family and friends played a large part in George's battle for survival. The extent of the prayer chain in place for his healing was beyond our comprehension at the time. Our next-door neighbor explored the Internet, intent on putting George's name on the Wailing Wall in Jerusalem. Our church congregation spoke his name in prayer each week. God heard many voices saying George's name that summer. Even now, years later, people we had not known at the time tell us that they remember praying for George.

Some people, though they may pray for someone they have been close to before serious illness became evident, will appear to avoid face-to-face contact. It if seems that a friend or family member has deserted you, the avoidance might be reasonably explained. Visitors sometimes feel uncomfortable around a person they believe to be in a terminal condition. I heard of one person afraid to visit someone with whom she had shared a long friendship, fearful that the friend might die in front of her eyes.

Many people harbor unanswered questions; hesitancy about what to talk about and how to act makes them stay away, and the person battling cancer is left with a sense of abandonment. People avoid those who are seriously ill for a number of reasons: fear of doing or saying the "wrong thing," uncertainty about how long to stay, worry over a correct topic of conversation. A potential visitor does not wish to sound too cheerful or too gloomy.

If the prognosis is not favorable, what should a visitor say? In our culture, many people find it difficult, if not impossible, to talk about candidly about death—their own or that of someone close. Consider the phrase, *if something should happen to.* The word *die* in this context is avoided, even the possible cost of hurting feelings. Death is associated with loss and grief and can resurrect forgotten memories that many would like to erase. All these issues are common and natural; many people inexperienced in hospital or home visiting harbor vague fears that make them avoid the seriously ill.

However, true friends can overcome such obstacles with the help of the sick person's caregiver—the best advocate in arranging for visits. Just as caregivers need to ask for help in coping with their own workload, they need to be direct in asking for visitors if their loved one wants company. Visitors need to keep the call short. Long pauses in conversation may be normal. Sick people aren't used to talking fast; brain tumor patients especially do not talk or think quickly. Often visitors can offer comfort and convey love and concern just by sitting quietly nearby. Their presence will be enough. Most of us are conditioned to saying or doing something in every situation. Sustained silence is not something we are always comfortable with.

Sick people tired easily and can become weary of the voices of even their closest friends. The give-and-take of normal conversation for those who are brain injured can be exhausting. Talking and listening require mental exercise that can sap one's small reservoir of energy. Visitors need to keep their remarks short and simple. There is a good chance that the patient would like to hear about something other than topics having to do with illness, even if there is no immediate response and the conversation appears to wane. Also, it is inappropriate for visitors to describe their own illnesses and symptoms.

I have visited patients who have pictures of their dogs or cats taped to the wall within easy view from the bed. Some health-care facilities allow pets to visit or even bring in volunteers with therapy dogs. Your loved one might enjoy a visit from a four-legged friend. Therapy dogs have to be newly bathed and brushed and their manners have to be impeccable—no barking or jumping. Our own dog stayed by George's side whenever he was home between chemotherapy infusions. Stroking a dog or cat has proven to be a great source of comfort for sick people.

There are alternatives to face-to-face visiting. Telephone calls are OK, if the patient is up to it, but conversations should be even shorter than visits in person. It's much better to send a card or a brief note addressed to the patient. Caregivers can read the notes to their loved ones at appropriate times. I have saved the notes and cards sent to George and will treasure them always.

When we interact with others in ways that show we care, we are sharing hope, much as Charles at the beginning of our cancer journey came to the hospital to share a message of hope. Charles did not react to George's appearance—the drooling mouth, the trembling hands, halting speech. He was not visibly shaken, nor did he offer false cheer. To tell an obviously ill person that he or she looks good is a blatant lie. To tell a terminally ill person that he is sure to survive is not an offer of hope but an act of cruelty.

Dr. Jerome Groopman, in *Anatomy of Hope: How People Prevail in the Face of Illness*, defines hope as a central force that keeps us strong in the face of adversity. Groopman is clear in his emphasis that there is difference between false hope and the absence of hope. False hope tries to offer something that does not exist. False hope is a lie.

True hope requires courage and strength. As I have wavered along this scary journey of my husband's brain cancer, someone was always there, ready to pick me up and offer the gift of hope. For George and me, it seems that hope and faith go together. Hope strengthens faith and faith upholds hope. We can do no less than try to pass on the gift of hope to others as it was given to us.

Throughout our brain tumor journey, we have seen the finest human qualities. Brain tumors, malignant and benign, are serious, life-changing diseases, and the people who survive them—for days or years—are living examples of bravery. We have mourned with those who suffer losses, and rejoiced with those who have been granted more time. For all whose lives have been touched with brain tumors or cancer of any sort, this book is for you.

David Bailey, the brain tumor survivor and folk singer, once wrote a poem about hope. Some day, he says, he might write the music for it as well, but for now he shares the words.

When

When you feel overwhelmed by the things you have to do
And you know you need to start but you haven't got a clue

When the hour hand is moving faster than it should
And you'd stop it in a second if you thought you could

When you wonder how on earth you'll make it through the day
And you feel like raising hell cuz heaven's just too far away

When anger and fatigue are running in your veins
And you're looking for the sun but the skies are full of rain

When every single breath feels like a chore
And the fears you thought were buried are knocking at your door

When every dream you built up is going down in smoke
And every prayer you whisper feels like a joke

When the friends you thought you trusted turn their backs and walk away
And you want to speak your mind but you don't know what to say

When you're trying to remember but you constantly forget
And you're hanging on to hope but you're haunted by regret

When you're trying to take it easy but everything is hard
And you want to find your freedom but always feel on guard
When every single sunset only makes you sad
And you want to just forgive but you can't stop being mad

When the questions keep on coming but the answers lag behind
And you're lost in the confusion of the fog inside your mind

When your heart is feeling heavy and spirit's feeling down
And the look upon your face is frozen in a frown

When you wish that you were proud but all you feel is shame
And you're hiding in the dark 'cause you cannot see the flame

When you wish you could rejoice but all you do is grieve
And you're seeking out your faith but you can't seem to believe

When the colors all around you fade to gray and then to black
And you put your best foot forward then retreat under attack

When you think everything's wrong and you're sure nothing is right
And you hold onto your vision but the end is out of sight

When the song you're trying to sing is quiet as the moon
And the star you wish upon falls away like a balloon

When it hurts too much to laugh 'cause all you do is cry
There's a reason to continue I will tell you why

If you are reading this it means you are not dead
And every breath you take and every thought inside your head

Is a crystal clear decree that God believes in you
And as long as you are here He's got more for you to do

And if per chance you stumble and fall upon the ground
And look in all directions but see no one around
It could be that everybody else has fallen too
And as much as you need them somebody else needs you

So rise up, my friend, and welcome this new day with a shout
Cherish every second and drive away the doubt

Walk right through the shadows, I promise there's a way
Then find out why the good Lord's given you another day.

—David M. Bailey, used with permission

Appendix A
Caregiver's Bill of Rights

I have the right ...

- to take care of myself. This is not an act of selfishness. It will give me the capability of taking better care of my loved one.

- to seek help from others even though others may object. I recognize the limits of my own strength and endurance.

- to maintain facets of my own life that do not include the person I care for, just as I would if he or she were healthy. I know that I do everything that I reasonable can for this person, and I have the right to do some things just for myself.

- to get angry, be depressed, and express other difficult feelings occasionally.

- to reject any attempts by my loved one (either conscious or unconscious) to manipulate me through guilt and/or depression.

- to receive consideration, affection, forgiveness, and acceptance from my loved one for what I do, for as long as I offer these qualities in return.

- to take pride in what I am accomplishing and to applaud the courage it has sometimes taken to meet the needs of my loved one.

- to protect my individuality and my right to make a life for myself that will sustain me in the time what my relative no longer needs my full-time help.

- to expect and demand that as new strides are made in finding resources to aid physically and mentally impaired persons in our country, similar strides will be made toward aiding and supporting caregivers.

—Author Unknown

Appendix B
Resources for Further Information

American Board of Clinical Neuropsychology
www.theabcn.org

American Board of Pediatric Neuropsychology
www.abpdn.org

American Brain Tumor Association
2720 River Road, Des Plaines, Illinois 60018
1-800-886-2282
www.abta.org

American Cancer Society
1-800-227-2345
www.cancer.org

Brain Injury Association
www.biausa.org

Brain Trust
www.braintrust.org
Offers online support groups.

Brain tumor stories and help
www.brainhospice.com
Includes a special place for caregivers to post their stories.

Brain Tumor Action Network
www.btan.org

Cancer Care
National Office, 275 Seventh Ave. New York, New York 10001
1-800-813-HOPE
www.cancercare.org

Cancer Counseling Inc.
www.cancerhouston.com

Cancer Information Service
1-800-4-CANCER
www.cis.nci.gov

Caregiver's Bill of Rights
www.mindspring.com

Central Brain Tumor Registry of the United States (CBTRUS)
www.cbtrus.org

Colorado Neurological Institute—CNI Center for Brain and Spinal Tumors
303-806-7420
www.TheCNI.org

David Bailey
www.Davidmbailey.com

Hospice Net
www.hospicenet.org

Leukemia and Lymphoma Society
1-800-955-4572
www.leukemia-lymphoma.org

MD Anderson Cancer Center
1515 Holcombe Blvd., Houston, TX 77030-4009
713-792-2121
www.mdanderson.org

National Brain Tumor Foundation
1-800-934-CURE
www.braintumor.org

National Cancer Institute
1-800-4-CANCER
www.cancer.gov

National Coalition for Cancer Survivorship
Offers a helpful free resource: The Cancer Survival Toolbox. This is a set
of nine modules that discuss all aspects of a cancer journey.
www.cancersurvivaltoolbox.org 1-877-866-5748

National Family Caregivers Association
1-800-896-3650
www.nfcacares.org

National Institute of Neurological Disorders and Stroke
www.ninds.nih.gov

National Organization of Social Security Claimants' Representatives
1-800-431-2804
www.nosscr.org

Neuropathy Association
www.neuropathy.org

North American Brain Tumor Coalition
www.nabraintumor.org

Oncology Channel
www.oncologychannel.com

Richard Bloch Cancer Foundation
1-800-433-0464/816-932-8453
www.blochcancer.com

Social Security
1-800-772-1213
www.ssa.gov

The Brain Tumor Society
1-800-770-8287
www.tbts.org

Today's Caregiver: A Magazine for Family and Professional Caregivers
6365 Taft Street, Suite 3003, Hollywood, FL 33024
www.caregiver.com

Appendix C
For Further Reading

Babcock, Elise NeeDell (founder of Cancer Counseling, Inc.). *When Life Becomes Precious: A Guide for Loved Ones and Friends of Cancer Patients.* New York: Bantam Books, 1997.

Brio, David. *One Hundred Days: My Unexpected Journey from Doctor to Patient.* New York: Random House, 2000.

Cooke, Robert C. *Dr. Folkman's War: Angiogenesis and the Struggle to Defeat Cancer.* New York: Random House, 2001.

Cousins, Norman. *Anatomy of an Illness: Reflections on Healing and Regeneration.* New York: W. Norton and Company, 1979.

——. *The Healing Heart: Antidotes to Panic and Helplessness.* W. W. Norton and Company, 1983.

Didier, Darryl C. *Force a Miracle.* Lincoln: iUniverse, 2002.

Dossey, Larry, M.D. *Prayer is Good Medicine: How to Reap the Healing Benefits of Prayer.* Harper: San Francisco, 1997.

——. *Healing Words: The Power and the Practice of Medicine.* San Francisco: Harper, 1993.

——. *Reinventing Medicine: Beyond Mind-Body to a New Era of Healing.* San Francisco: Harper, 1993.

Groopman, Jerome, M.D. *The Anatomy of Hope: How People Prevail in the Face of Illness.* New York: Random House, 2004.

Holzemer, Liz. *Curveball: When Life Throws You a Brain Tumor.* Ghost Road Press, 2007

Klein, Allen. *The Healing Power of Humor: Techniques for Getting Through Loss, Setbacks, Upsets, Disappointments, Difficulties, Trials, Tribulations, and All That Not-So-Funny Stuff.* Los Angeles: Jeremy Tarcher, Inc., 1989.

Kushner, Harold S. *When Bad Things Happen to Good People.* New York: Schoken Books, 1981.

L'Engle, Madeleine. *Two-Part Invention: The Story of a Marriage.* San Francisco: Harper and Row, 1989.

Moyers, Bill. *Healing and the Mind.* New York: Doubleday, 1993.

Raver Lampman, Greg. *Magic and Loss.* Hampton Roads Publishing, 1994.

Smith, Gregory, and Steven Naifeh. *Making Miracles Happen.* Boston: Little, Brown, and Company, 1997.

Stoler, Diane Roberts, Ed.D., and Barbara Albers Hill. *Coping with Mild Traumatic Brain Injury: A Guide to Living with the Challenges Associated with Concussion/Brain Injury.* City: Avery, 1998.

Glossary of Terms

Aphasia Loss of the use of language. Expressive aphasia affects speech. Receptive aphasia affects ability to understand speech.

Ataxia Impaired ability to coordinate movement shown by a staggering gait and disturbed sense of balance.

Benign Tumor Does not invade surrounding tissues or metastasize in other sites. Its cells are not generally malignant.

Blood-Brain Barrier Prevents or slows the passage of chemical compounds such as chemotherapy drugs from the blood into the central nervous system.

Calcium Leukovorin Given after the chemotherapy drug Methotrexate and acts to stop its toxic effects. Also called Wellcovorin, the medicine acts as a "rescue" to prevent Methotrexate from going beyond killing cancer cells, causing life threatening toxicity to your bone marrow, mouth, and gastro-intestinal tract.

Clinical Trials Research studies in which people participate. Clinical trials may be conducted by a single institution or by several institutions acting as a single unit. Strict standards and supervision govern clinical trials. Drugs such as Temozolomide (Temodor) were tested in clinical trials and are now widely used in treating brain cancer.

Decadron A corticosteroid, similar to a natural hormone produced by your adrenal glands. It is used to manage certain severe allergic conditions, asthma, certain forms of arthritis, and skin, eye, thyroid, blood, and intestinal disorders. The drug was given to George to manage the swelling of the tumor and the surrounding areas in the brain. Other names are Dexamethasone, Dexone, Hexafrol, Mymethasone.

Lymphoma Also called **CNS Lymphoma** or **Primary CNS lymphoma (PCL).** Affects those with malfunctioning immune systems, but is increasing in people with healthy immune systems. This lymphoma is most commonly B-cell, non-Hodgkin's type.

Meningioma The most prevalent type of benign brain tumor. Because it is slow growing, it can grow become large before symptoms become obvious. If the tumor is accessible, the standard treatment is surgery to remove it. Radiation is sometimes required as well. A subtype is **atypical meningioma,** faster growing with a tendency to spread and recur.

Metastatic Brain Tumor A tumor formed by cancer cells that have spread from another part of the body. For example, lung cancer cells that spread to the brain are still defined as lung cancer. Other sites of origin for metastatic brain tumors are the skin, breast, and colon. All metastatic tumors are malignant.

Needle Biopsy A surgical procedure where a small hole is drilled into the skull, and then a needle is inserted. Tissue is removed from the core of the needle and sent to the pathologist.

Neuro Oncologist A doctor with training both in neurology and in oncology (cancer).

Neuropsychologist A psychologist specializing on the relation between brain and behavior. Neuropsychologists help brain tumor survivors determine the way they learn and cope best, and design programs to maximize survivors' strengths as part of living style.

Ommaya Reservoir A small "container" surgically placed under the scalp with a tube leading into a section of the brain. Medications are injected via syringe into the reservoir to deliver chemotherapy drugs directly into the cerebrospinal fluid, bathing the brain and spinal cord with the drugs.

PICC (Peripherally Inserted Central Catheter) One type of catheter used to administer medications or blood products and to be able to draw blood for tests. The catheter is a small plastic tube (made of silicone) placed in a vein in your arm and threaded into a large vein near the entrance to your heart. There may be sutures (stitches) securing the catheter to the skin.

Platelets The blood cells that prevent or stop bleeding. Anticancer drugs can affect the body's production of blood cells in the bone marrow. If your platelet count gets too low, you may have symptoms such as bruising or bleeding.

Primary Malignant Brain Tumor A tumor whose origin is in the brain.

Protocol A written plan specifying the procedures to be followed in providing for a particular condition. Also called a plan of care.

Stereotaxic Biopsy A computer directed needle biopsy. The computer, using information from a CY or MRI scan, provides precise information about a tumor's location.

About the Author

Ann Brandt holds a BA and MA in English. She is a member of Colorado Authors' League and Denver Women's Press Club.

Experiencing serious disease from two viewpoints has given Ann a unique perspective on coping with life-changing issues. One year into recovery from Guillain Barre, Ann found herself in the role of caregiver when her husband was diagnosed with primary CNS non-Hodgkin's lymphoma, a rare form of brain cancer. Calling upon her memories of being cared for the previous year, she resolved to be "the best caregiver I could be."

During a battle with brain tumors, caregivers' needs can take second place. Ann believes that support groups are often the best emotional support available for people caring for brain tumor patients. She attends her husband's support group meetings, talking with caregivers and patients.

Remembering her own experience with life-changing disease, Ann serves as liaison for the Guillain Barre Foundation International, based in Pennsylvania. She visits patients in hospitals and rehabilitation centers, counsels families, and organizes support group meetings.

Ann has written and published numerous articles and essays for national and local publications, including the *Chicken Soup for the Soul* series. She and her husband George live in Broomfield, Colorado with their large, furry canine companion, Lucky, who was caregiver for both of her owners.

978-0-595-44883-8
0-595-44883-6